Secrets of Success
Getting into GP Training

Secrets of Success
Getting into GP Training

Edited by

Jasdeep Gill MBChB(Hons), DRCOG, DFSRH
ST2 in General Practice, London Deanery,
London, UK

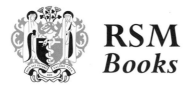
RSM
Books

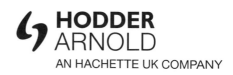
HODDER
ARNOLD
AN HACHETTE UK COMPANY

First published in Great Britain in 2010 by
Hodder Arnold, an imprint of Hodder Education, an Hachette UK company,
338 Euston Road, London NW1 3BH

http://www.hodderarnold.com

Hachette Livre UK's policy is to use papers that are natural, renewable and recyclable
products and made from wood grown in sustainable forests. The logging and
manufacturing processes are expected to conform to the environmental regulations of
the country of origin.

Whilst the advice and information in this book are believed to be true and accurate at
the date of going to press, neither the author[s] nor the publisher can accept any legal
responsibility or liability for any errors or omissions that may be made. In particular,
(but without limiting the generality of the preceding disclaimer) every effort has
been made to check drug dosages; however it is still possible that errors have been
missed. Furthermore, dosage schedules are constantly being revised and new side-
effects recognized. For these reasons the reader is strongly urged to consult the drug
companies' printed instructions before administering any of the drugs recommended
in this book.

British Library Cataloguing in Publication Data
A catalogue record for this book is available from the British Library

Library of Congress Cataloging-in-Publication Data
A catalog record for this book is available from the Library of Congress

ISBN 978 1 853 15954 1

1 2 3 4 5 6 7 8 9 10

Commissioning Editor: Caroline Makepeace
Project Editor: Joanna Silman
Production Controller: Kate Harris
Cover Design: Lynda King
Indexer: Lisa Footit

Cover image © Getty Images

The logo of the Royal Society of Medicine is a registered trade mark, which it has
licensed to Hodder Arnold.

What do you think about this book? Or any other Hodder Arnold title?
Please visit our website: www.hodderarnold.com

Typeset in Scotland by IMH(Cartrif), EH20 9DX
Printed and bound in the UK by Antony Rowe

Contents

Contributors

Jasdeep Gill MBChB (Hons), DRCOG, DFSRH
ST2 in General Practice, London Deanery, UK

Anthea Lints MBChB, FRCGP, MCliSci
Director of Postgraduate General Practice Education, South East
Scotland Deanery, UK

Rajesh Kumar MBChB
ST2 in General Practice, East Midlands Deanery, UK

Annabelle MacGregor MBBS, MRCPCH, MA, Grad(Dip) Law
ST3 in General Practice, London Deanery, UK

Sukhjinder Nijjer MBChB (Hons), BSc (Hons), MRCP,
Academic Clinical Fellow in Cardiology, London Deanery, UK

Foreword

A General Practitioner is a specialist trained to provide frontline and continuous health care to a practice population, and to individual patients and their families, across a spectrum of preventative care and illness which encompasses physical, psychological, social and occupational factors.

The aims and objectives of the GP recruitment and selection system (i.e. the gateway to entry into general practice specialty training) embrace both the desire to attract the brightest and best doctors into the specialty and also to ensure, through a valid, reliable and fair selection process, that successful applicants have the necessary knowledge, skills and attitudes to train as general practitioners.

Quite apart from ensuring clinical competence during the GP training programme, future GPs must also be 'fit for purpose' through the acquisition of leadership and management skills, the ability to work in multiprofessional teams and to manage their work life balance in the modern NHS.

Given the policy context of a primary care led NHS and professionally led commissioning of patient care by GPs, there is also an increasing need to invest in appropriate GP workforce planning and the future development of the GP workforce.

Being a GP is a rewarding and challenging experience. It is also an exciting time to choose general practice as a career pathway and this book provides expert and helpful step-by-step guidance into general practice specialty training.

Professor Neil Jackson
Dean of Postgraduate General Practice Education,
London Deanery

Acknowledgements

With thanks to the GP National Recruitment Office and Dr John Gillies for their kind assistance and permission granted for material in this book.

With thanks to the contributors and everyone at Hodder Education, particularly Caroline Makepeace, Francesca Naish and Joanna Silman, for their hard work and cooperation.

With special thanks to Sarah Ogden and Peter Richardson at the Royal Society of Medicine for their support at the start of this project.

This book is dedicated to all the upcoming doctors keen to join this unique specialty - best of luck!

List of abbreviations used

AAA	abdominal aortic aneurysm
ACF	Academic Clinical Fellowship
ARCP	Annual Review of Competence Progression
ARDS	acute respiratory distress syndrome
BMI	body mass index
BTS	British Thoracic Society
BV	bacterial vaginosis
CCT	Certificate of Completion of Training
CDH	congenital dislocation of the hip
CKD	chronic kidney disease
COPD	chronic obstructive pulmonary disease
CPAP	continuous positive airway pressure
CPD	continuous professional development
CPR	cardiopulmonary resuscitation
CRP	C-reactive protein
CSF	cerebrospinal fluid
CT	computed tomography
DEN	doctor's educational need
DKA	diabetic ketoacidosis
DVLA	Driver and Vehicle Licensing Agency
EBV	Epstein–Barr virus
FACD	Foundation Achievement of Competence Document
FPO	Foundation Programme Office
GMC	General Medical Council
GP	General practitioner
GPST	GP specialty training
HDL	high-density lipoprotein
HDU	high dependency unit

IBS	Irritable bowel syndrome
IELTS	International English Language and Testing System
IUS	intrauterine system
LINks	local involvement networks
LTFTT	less than full-time training
LTOT	long-term oxygen therapy
MAHA	microangiopathic haemolytic anaemia
MAU	medical assessment unit
MCV	mean corpuscular volume
MI	myocardial infarction
MMSE	Mini Mental State Examination
MRI	magnetic resonance imaging
MS	multiple sclerosis
MST	morphine sulphate tablets
NBM	nil by mouth
NHS	National Health Service
NICE	National Institute of Health and Clinical Excellence
NPS	National Person Specification
NRO	National Recruitment Office
OCP	oral contraceptive pill
OGTT	oral glucose tolerance test
PALS	Patient Advice and Liaison Services
PCA	patient-controlled analgesia
PCI	percutaneous coronary intervention
PCOS	polycystic ovary syndrome
PE	pulmonary embolus
PEA	pulseless electrical activity
PEFR	peak expiratory flow rate
PLAB	Professional and Linguistic Assessment Board
PMETB	Postgraduate Medical Education Training Board
PSA	prostate-specific antigen
PUN	patient's unmet need
QOF	Quality and Outcomes Framework
SJT	situational judgement test
SLE	systemic lupus erythematosus
SPECT	single photon emission computed tomography
STEMI	ST segment elevation myocardial infarction
STI	sexually transmitted infections
SUFE	slipped upper femoral epiphysis
TB	tuberculosis
TIA	transient ischaemic attack
TOP	termination of pregnancy
UKMEC	UK Medical Eligibility Criteria
WHO	World Health Organization

Key for Icons

 Top Tip

 Danger

 Question

 Ask the Expert

 Facts and Figures

 Homework

SECTION A

Applying for general practice specialty training

1 Introduction to general practice

Anthea Lints and Jasdeep Gill

Evolution and change in general practice

General practice forms a crucial part of medical care in the UK. General practitioners (GPs) are the first port of call and gatekeepers to specialist services within the NHS. They have a privileged role and responsibility within the community to serve and safeguard their patients.

In recent years, general practice and general practice training in the UK have undergone major changes. Despite frequent bureaucratic shifts and increasing service pressure, general practice remains a vibrant and exciting prospect for young doctors embarking on their specialty career.

Historically, it would seem that 'general practitioners' have been around at least since the early nineteenth century following the passage of the Apothecaries Act. Medicine at that time was dominated by the powerful Royal Colleges of Medicine and Surgery. It was not until 1952 that the College of General Practitioners was established and described as 'an outstanding event in the history of British medicine'. In 1972, the college acquired its Royal Charter and mandatory training was required for all new GPs. Since then, the Health Service has seen many dramatic policy changes including an internal NHS market and GP fund holding (1991–7), the NHS Plan (2000) and Our Health, Our Care, Our Say which saw the reintroduction of competition and private service provision in the NHS in 2005.

General practice has remained resilient, rising to the challenges imposed upon it. In training, we have seen a new curriculum, new assessments and a new RCGP examination. The current GMS contract which includes the Quality and Outcomes Framework (QOF) is largely evidence based. Recent political changes meant that four different health economies are emerging from the devolved nations each with different priorities and frameworks to deliver health care to those for whom they are responsible.

It is evident that the future of general practice is secure provided future GPs are willing to embrace the key roles which are evolving as a consequence of service changes. These key roles are summarized, with permission from the authors,[1] in the following box:

- Generalist
- Chronic disease management
- Prevention of ill health
- Teaching colleagues/self
- Team working
- Holistic/personal care
- Continuity/coordinated care

What makes a good GP?

This is one of those philosophical questions that depends upon the definition of 'good'. In *Distilling the essence of general practice: a learning journey in progress*[1] Gillies et al. identify the qualities required of a GP in the future as including the following:

- robust intellect/passion for knowledge
- altruism and commitment
- awareness of justice
- integrity
- respect for patients
- empathy/emotional awareness
- capacity for innovation
- ability to work with others.

The development of a competency model for general practice was initially conducted via a job analysis in the late 1990s and then published in the *British Journal of General Practice* in 2000.[2] This provided the blueprint and decision-making platform for the design, implementation and validation of short listing and selection centre methodologies for the GP National Recruitment Office. The original GP job analysis has been the cornerstone to the successful GP selection process. The national GP specialty training entry process is assessed against the GP Person Specification which is detailed in Chapter 4. The current GP selection system has proven to be effective and robust through a difficult period in medical selection.[3] It is recognized by many as the 'gold standard' in medical selection.

Why choose general practice?

It can be daunting to select a career pathway and commit to several years of training and subsequent career. Think carefully about where you see yourself in 5 to 10 years and indeed beyond that. There are a number of resources designed to help doctors in training reach a decision with which they feel comfortable. Many deaneries offer career advice and mentoring schemes. Many doctors can undertake a 'taster' period in the specialty in which they are interested. These resources are designed to help trainees decide whether a career in general practice would suit their personality and aspirations.

General practice is a unique specialty. It is a discipline in which the doctor–patient relationship is the active ingredient of almost everything that is achieved.[4] It also encapsulates the need for teamwork, management and business skills alongside the art of clinical acumen. In 2007, the Royal College of General Practitioners defined the curriculum, based on *Being a general practitioner* which describes 75 learning outcomes for GP trainees. The key advantages and essence of general practice are described by Gillies et al. below.[1]

- **Trust:** achieved by high-quality empathic communication with patients and past experience of good-quality care,[5] essential for concordance with treatment, co-creation of health, effective gate keeping and avoidance of medicalization. Underpinned by local perceptions of altruism, fair dealing and other personal qualities, competence, integrity and probity and by both rhetoric and an assumption of good intentions.[6]

- **Coordination:** in dealing with patients' multiple problems and issues: between patients and relatives/partners, between GP and members of the primary healthcare team, social work and voluntary agencies, between hospital consultant-led and primary care services.

- **Continuity:** generated by repeated contacts, developing and strengthening relationships with patients over months and years. Challenged by many trends, including the feminization of general practice and new working patterns among GPs, including daytime working, multiple providers of care and GP-led health centres.

- **Flexibility:** to address problems in the order and at a pace that suits patients: adapting clinical evidence to the individual patient; GMS contract requirements to local community needs; balancing individual and population approaches in day-to-day work; dealing capably with continuing NHS change; liaising effectively with local voluntary organizations and innovating to good effect.

- **Coverage:** comprising over 90% contact with list populations over a 5-year period, including many who are 'hard to reach' using one-off screening approaches so that special measures to enhance coverage are required for very few people. This cumulative approach to population coverage is much more sustainable than screening.

- **Leadership:** including the ability to implement change quickly, based on multidisciplinary knowledge and experience of local circumstances, staffing and population characteristics.

The highs and lows

The working life of a GP is variable and flexible. This is not only in their daily practice but throughout their career. Most GPs are able to effectively combine their clinical work with other interests and commitments. Some GPs choose to work as salaried GPs and others prefer the additional responsibilities and risks associated with partnership.

Every day brings unexpected challenges. Here are a few memorable moments from the clinical career of one GP:

Mr A, who worked in the photographic industry, had escaped the Nazi invasion of Poland and made a successful career in England. He presented with breathlessness and lack of energy and was diagnosed soon after presentation with an extensive mesothelioma. Treatment at best was considered unlikely to prolong his life by anything more than a few painful months and instead he chose to revisit favourite places across Europe with his wife who was entirely supportive of his wishes. In his final few weeks, an attempt to include the local hospice in his care was rejected on the grounds that he perceived the organization was too concerned with his soul. I visited daily until his death. He invited all who had been involved in his care individually and by appointment to share a glass of excellent wine and when all had gone simply whispered 'poof, puff' to his devoted wife and drifted into a painless coma.

An 11-year-old boy presented with the typical symptoms of a sore throat in the midst of winter when upper respiratory infections dominated most consultations. His mother whom I knew well seemed extraordinarily concerned, which was unusual. There was something that simply did not sit comfortably and a blood test which was not something I would normally have requested so early in the natural history of a sore throat, revealed leukaemia. He responded well to treatment.

On call, the phone rang at 2 a.m. A father some 10 miles away demanded an immediate house call to treat his 5-year-old daughter whom he had discovered had head lice. It was clear the request was not debateable. It was shortly after, that the Department of Health renegotiated the GP contract which allowed GPs to opt out of providing 24-hour care to their patients, a service which had sadly been eroded and abused over the years.

An average day in the life of a GP

6.30 a.m. The alarm clock on the radio heralds a new day. Up, shower, dress and eat, while encouraging children to do same.

7.30 a.m. Drive children to school 8 miles in the opposite direction to the surgery, while traffic steadily building up to its rush hour crescendo.

8.30 a.m. Arrive in surgery, quick coffee while reception staff rapidly fill appointments (if they keep coming in at this rate I'm doomed).

8.40 a.m. Log on to computer, quick scan through messages and 'to do' list.

9.00 a.m. Surgery starts and apparently I have an aspirational coffee break at 10.30 a.m. Our surgery involves walking along a corridor to collect patients from the waiting room which allows for a few informal brief conversations with colleagues en route and the added benefit of interpatient exercise and potential weight control. Usual run of minor ailments interspersed with some more potentially serious symptoms which will need further investigation. Sometimes the surgery is interrupted by:

- a nurse or trainee who needs advice
- a receptionist who wants to add a few extras to my list

- a request for an emergency visit, for example to coax a child with behaviour problems off the roof where she is sitting with fire brigade and police in attendance.

This last request means neither coffee nor lunch.

1 p.m. Return to surgery with child no longer on roof but in care of Child and Adolescent Services to whom she is well known, hence co-operation assured.

Have been allocated a visit to an elderly patient who has 'gone off her legs'.

1.15 p.m. Phone elderly patient who has 'gone off her legs' and establish she is fed, warm and safe for time being so can wait until I have completed essential paperwork from morning surgery which was completed abruptly.

1.30 p.m. Join lunchtime clinical meeting with primary healthcare team, including health visitors and district nurses, which in the current climate we are lucky to have, then meeting with practice manager to discuss organizational and managerial issues.

2.00 p.m. Visit patient who has indeed 'gone off her legs', followed by hide and seek exercise in attempt to contact local social services. Their phone is constantly engaged – they must be very busy.

3.00 p.m. Follow-up visit to patient with motor neurone disease who has been set up with a respirator and feeling generally happier. He desperately wants to give his daughter away when she gets married next month – he should make it.

4.00 p.m. Time to start evening surgery which happens to be relatively straightforward.

6.30 p.m. Have finished afternoon surgery and checked through results, prescriptions and correspondence for the day. The out of hours provider takes over responsibility. Wind down by chatting with colleagues who have also finished their surgeries and simply want to chat idly about life, the universe, the weekend and their families.

Types of general practice

Contractual obligations and the Quality Outcome Framework dictates much of what is expected by the Department of Health be delivered in primary care. Differences between practices are mostly in relation to demographics and geography. Large inner cities tend to be multicultural. One practice in the East End of London has calculated more than 70 languages represented by their patients. Chronic disease is aligned with deprivation, while the most affluent are often the most challenging and demanding. After training, choice of practice is dictated by a number of factors both personal and situational. While in the past, a general practitioner would remain in one practice for the entirety of his/her working life, this is no longer the case, and it is quite common and acceptable to move from one practice to another as circumstances dictate.

Employment options

Again, this is dictated by personal and situational factors. It used to be the aspiration of most trainees to acquire a profit-sharing partnership in what is essentially a small business. Now it is equally common for both male and female GPs to choose to work part time or as assistants where the administrative and managerial burden is often less. For those returning after a significant gap, UK deaneries offer returner schemes and for those with domestic commitments it is possible to do a limited amount of clinical work supported educationally by a mentor as part of the retainer scheme. Many GPs are self-constructing a portfolio career which may incorporate specific clinical interests and managerial, educational, advisory or leadership roles within other NHS organizations, for example, deaneries, primary care organizations, health boards or the Department of Health. There are options open to you in your career as a GP in addition to clinical commitments.

In summary, general practice is a unique specialty which offers doctors endless opportunity to utilize their clinical, personal and business skills. GPs play a vital role in the primary care of their patients from birth to the end of life. General practice is a challenging yet rewarding specialty and offers exciting evolving prospects to all doctors keen to embark on a career in general practice.

References

1. Gillies JCM, Mercer SW, Lyon A et al. Distilling the essence of general practice: A learning journey in progress. *Br J Gen Pract* 2009; **59**: 356–63.
2. Patterson F, Ferguson E, Lane P et al. A competency model for general practice: Implications for selection and development. *Br J Gen Pract* 2000; **50**: 188–93.
3. Plint S, Patterson F. The way forward for recruitment into specialty training in the UK: Identifying critical success factors. *Postgrad Med J* 2010; **86**: 323–7.
4. McWhinney I. The importance of being different. The Pickles Lecture. *Br J Gen Pract* 1996; **46**: 433–6.
5. Tarrant C, Colman A, Stokes T. Past experience 'shadow of the future' and patient trust: A cross-sectional survey. *Br J Gen Pract* 2008; **58**: 780–3.
6. Freidson E. *Professionalism: The third logic. On the practice of knowledge.* Chicago, Il.: University of Chicago Press, 2001.

2 Introduction to GP specialty training

Anthea Lints

The start of GP training

General practice training became mandatory for all GPs in 1972. Before then it was possible to start working as a GP following house jobs with no training specifically for or in primary care. After 1972, a small number of trainees entered 3-year managed GP vocational training programmes, while others constructed their own programme with a mixture of hospital-based posts and 12 months in the general practice setting as a GP trainee.

The regulations were very liberal and allowed trainees with very narrow previous experience to simply complete training with 12 months in practice. On the other hand, it encouraged free spirit and career change. Until 2000, recruitment to GP trainee posts was generally arranged locally.

In 2000, these arrangements were dramatically changed, when deaneries were required to manage recruitment to ensure equality of opportunity and the selection of those trainees best suited to the specialty. The directors of postgraduate general practice education agreed that the process should be co-ordinated nationally through the GP National Recruitment Office to professionalize the recruitment process and to ensure consistency across the UK.

In 2007, the changes to medical training, implemented through the Modernising Medical Careers agenda, meant that GP specialist training, leading to a Certificate of Completion of Training (CCT), could only be secured through a managed programme approved by the PMETB (Postgraduate Medical Education Training Board) for a minimum of 3 years. In addition, the RCGP designed a curriculum, an assessment framework and an electronic portfolio. Until 2010, the regulatory body was PMETB whose responsibility was to approve specialty curriculum and assessment processes which included a system of educational and clinical supervision and annual review of competency progression. These changes have mostly been welcome and have improved the quality of training, training programmes and the trainee experience. The PMETB ceased to exist in March 2010, but their regulatory and operational frameworks have been adopted by the General Medical Council (GMC) which has, since April 2010, become the regulator for all medical training within the UK.

Pathway to becoming a GP

Many would say that the pathway to becoming a GP starts at medical school. Most UK medical schools have a strong element of general practice teaching within their curriculum. The most conventional pathway into GP specialty training for UK graduates is to apply for a GP specialty training (GPST) programme during FY2 (foundation year 2), as illustrated in Figure 2.1. Some foundation programmes have a general practice placement within the rotation. This can give you a useful insight into general practice. However, it is not essential and is not a requirement for applying to GP specialty training. For those who have not done a UK foundation programme, there are other means of proving acquisition of foundation competencies that would confer eligibility to apply for a GPST programme.

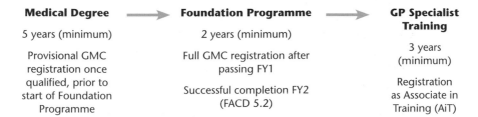

Medical Degree	**Foundation Programme**	**GP Specialist Training**
5 years (minimum)	2 years (minimum)	3 years (minimum)
Provisional GMC registration once qualified, prior to start of Foundation Programme	Full GMC registration after passing FY1 Successful completion FY2 (FACD 5.2)	Registration as Associate in Training (AiT)

Figure 2.1 Conventional pathway into GP training

For doctors who have trained abroad, it is possible to submit equivalent experience to the GMC for consideration of certification under Article 11. Details of this route can be found on the RCGP website within the section describing the requirements for certification.

Entry to a GMC-approved GPST programme and successful completion of all the exams and assessments required leads to a CCT which enables independent practice as a GP in the UK.

Currently, most deaneries have 3-year GP specialist training programmes, however, there are a few 4-year training programmes available. In addition, there are some 4-year Academic Clinical Fellowship (ACF) posts for GP specialist training across the UK.

Those involved in training believe that 3 years is too short. Although trainees completing training are competent they are not confident to embark on independent practice. General practice is the shortest specialty training programme and this is only possible because of the close relationship between trainee and trainer. Where training capacity in primary care is stretched, the trainee experience inevitably suffers.

A survey of GP trainees in 2006 produced some surprising results. When asked what they would like included in their training programmes, the majority wanted more hospital-based training encompassing many more specialties which would have amounted to 44 months in hospital-based specialties.

The RCGP would like training programmes to be 5 years of which at least 2 and possibly 3 would be embedded in primary care. This would enable training to be more closely aligned to the needs of the service with GPs developing advanced skills to co-ordinate patient pathways and more community-based care plans. Before this can happen, the government need to be convinced that the additional financial investment would bring added measurable benefit.

At present, some deaneries are piloting longer programmes – some include additional training in hospital, while others include 24 months based in general practice. Evaluation of these programmes will influence future decisions. It would seem logical that training for general practice should be firmly embedded in a general practice setting. An extended period of training would allow consolidation of core learning and enable the acquisition of additional skills in research, audit, organization, management, teaching and leadership.

Normally programmes include a variety of 4- or 6-month hospital-based posts that would possibly include paediatrics, obstetrics, gynaecology, emergency medicine, general medicine, care of the elderly, psychiatry and palliative care, and some might include specialties, such as ophthalmology, ENT, rehabilitation medicine, dermatology and public health. Clearly, it is impossible for every trainee to gain experience within each of these specialties but most can be gained within the primary care setting and many would suggest that, for example, training in primary care paediatrics is more relevant when acquired within the GP training practice. Even hospital-based posts that do not appear an obvious choice within a GPST programme can be invaluable in developing skills relevant to general practice.

Less than full-time training

Although a part-time career in general practice is rewarding and feasible, part-time training is much more difficult. The effect of the European Working Time Directive and Borders Agency restrictions means that gaps in programmes created by part-time training and other unpredictable circumstances in hospital-based posts can no longer be filled. This has a consequential negative impact on training for the remaining full-time trainees. At present, part-time training in the general practice-based component of training is easier to support, but even those opportunities may in future be limited by funding. Each deanery manages less than full-time training (LTFTT) requests individually and guidelines can be found on deanery websites.

The RCGP curriculum

'Being a general practitioner', the core statement of the RCGP curriculum, contains 75 learning outcomes for GP trainees.[1,2]

These learning outcomes can be measured and assessed. In spite of this broad curriculum, there are elements of general practice that can be neither measured nor assessed. This has been referred to as the hidden curriculum.

Assessments during GP specialty training

It has been said that 'assessment drives learning', but trainees struggling to complete the required assessments do not always believe the adage. Figure 2.2 is a simplified diagram, illustrating the key components which must be successfully obtained during your GP specialty training programme to achieve the MRCGP. Information about the assessments are frequently updated on the RCGP website.

A certificate of completion of training (CCT) requires that all the necessary exams and assessments have been successfully completed and signed off by the deanery's ARCP (Annual Review of Competence Progression) panel.

Expectations of trainees

Deaneries, employers and patients expect trainees to comply with the professional standards described by the GMC in Good

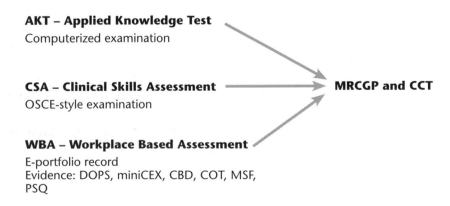

AKT – Applied Knowledge Test
Computerized examination

CSA – Clinical Skills Assessment
OSCE-style examination

MRCGP and CCT

WBA – Workplace Based Assessment
E-portfolio record
Evidence: DOPS, miniCEX, CBD, COT, MSF, PSQ

Figure 2.2 The key components which must be successfully obtained during GP specialty training programme to achieve the MRCGP.

Medical Practice.[3] In addition, GP specialty trainees are expected to:

- demonstrate exemplary professional standards
- observe the highest standards in relation to patient safety
- commit both clinically and educationally to their programme
- engage with the e-portfolio and submit the necessary assessments in a timely fashion
- prepare adequately for assessments, exams and the ARCP process
- strive to achieve more than the bare minimum required
- be prepared to give honest feedback to the regulator and to the deanery to enable improvement
- be mindful of the personal and professional needs of their fellow trainees.

In summary, GP training programmes are currently undergoing change. However, GP specialty training remains innovative and stimulating. It offers you the opportunity to be mentored closely and share your experiences with your peers and trainer. You will not only develop as a clinician, but also on a personal level. GP specialty training may seem a long way off at the moment, but this chapter will have given you insight into what it is likely to involve.

References

1. Royal College of General Practitioners. Being a general practitioner. Curriculum statement 1. London: RCGP Publications, 2007.
2. Riley B, Haynes J, Field S. *The condensed curriculum guide for GP training and the new MRCGP*. London: Royal College of General Practitioners, 2007.
3. General Medical Council. Good medical practice: Guidance for doctors. Effective from November 13, 2006. London: GMC.

SECTION B

GP specialty training entry process

3 The four-stage entry process

Jasdeep Gill

Introduction

This chapter will give you an overview of the entry process at a glance, with greater detail and advice given in the chapters to follow.

Recruitment into GP training is managed centrally on behalf of all the UK deaneries by the GP National Recruitment Office (NRO). The GP entry process involves four stages, which have been designed to assess an applicant's ability to fulfil the GP person specification.

The four stages of the GP specialty training entry process are summarized below. You must pass each stage of the entry process to proceed to the next. The GP NRO will notify you via email.

Following assessment, successful applicants will be offered GP specialty training programmes and they must accept or decline the offer within 48 hours. A system of local and national clearing is conducted, to help all suitable applicants obtain a training programme somewhere in the UK. A 'round 2' of all remaining GPST programmes is conducted which acts as a national clearing system. Refer to Chapter 14 to find out more about the clearing system.

Summary of GP specialty training entry process

Stage	Process	Recruitment calendar[a]
Stage 1: Long listing	Eligibility On-line application Rank 4 deanery preferences Proof of evidence	November
Stage 2: Short listing	Situational judgement test	Early January, across venues nationwide
Stage 3: Selection centre	Simulation exercise	From February, ensure your place is booked in advance
	Written prioritization exercise	
Stage 4: Offer/allocation	Offers emailed out	March, with 48 hours given to accept offer
	Local and national clearing	March and April

[a]Approximate based on 2011 – always check official dates on the GP training recruitment website.

Competition

Entry into GP specialty training is highly competitive. Despite frequent bureaucratic shifts and increasing service pressure, general practice remains a very popular, vibrant and exciting prospect for young doctors embarking on their specialty career. Remember, you will be competing against foundation year 2 doctors and more senior doctors from the UK and overseas who have chosen general practice as the career for them. The assessments are set at a level expected from that of foundation year 2 doctors.

The numbers of doctors applying to GPST programmes have risen steadily since 2000, although for entry in August 2010 the applications remained much the same as in the previous year, with an average competition ratio of 1:2. Competition ratios for each deanery can vary from year to year and can vary between stages. Choosing the deaneries in which you want to work can be a difficult and stressful decision. You will need to rank up to four deaneries in preference order early in the application process. The figures shown below are based on application to first choice deanery preferences.

Figures of national deanery vacancies 2010 (approximate) and competition ratios 2010

Deanery	Vacancies, 2010	Applicant:vacancy ratio, 2010
East of England	278	1.28
East Midlands	252	1.40
Kent, Surrey and Sussex	286	1.27
London	315	3.70
Mersey	142	1.40
Northern	156	1.56
Northern Ireland	65	2.92
Northwestern	255	1.87
Oxford	100	1.81
Scotland	320	1.28
Severn	126	1.60
Southwest peninsula	102	1.33
Wales	136	1.20
Wessex	145	1.15
West Midlands	318	1.74
Yorkshire and Humberside	309	1.39

Adapted from www.gprecruitment.org.uk

A guide to UK deanery profiles for GP training

This section aims to give you a consolidated overview of the UK deanery profiles for GP training. It is not an exhaustive guide, but serves as a key reference point prior to making your choices. Details regarding geographical location and programmes have been included, as well as the website link you should visit to find out more about the deaneries you are interested in. You should look closely at the geographical boundaries of your potential deaneries, because you may not initially realize that several deaneries could have a programme close to where you want to be. There is an exciting range of opportunities available at each deanery. You should explore the GP training programmes within the four deaneries you rank.

The information within this section is not biased by any personal opinion. It is presented to you in alphabetical order in an objective and systematic way. It would be sensible for you to try discussing the area and programme that you are interested in with colleagues or trainees within the programme to get a real sense of what it is like.

Ultimately, your decision of which four deaneries to rank and in which order will be based on a combination of factors, for example, geographical, financial, deanery reputation, family, schools for children – the list could go on. Some of these factors will be fixed and outside your control, whereas others may be variable. At this stage, it can be difficult to weigh up such decisions as to where the next 3 or more years of your training should be. However, it is crucial that you devote some time to considering your options and choosing deaneries which satisfy your individual needs.

Once you have made up to four deanery preferences, your application will be dealt with by your first choice deanery. If successful at stage 1, you will sit your stage 2 assessment within that deanery. Depending on the result of your stage 2 assessment, you will be allocated to a deanery for the stage 3 selection centre. Not all applicants will get their first choice deanery, so it is important that you select deaneries in which you are willing to work should the need arise. Remember that each deanery has a generally high standard of teaching and trainees are well supported, so do not be disheartened if you do not get your first choice.

When you attend for the stage 3 selection centre at your allocated deanery, you may be asked to rank the programmes in preference order. Most deaneries send you the programme ranking information beforehand, whereas some request it on the day. It is essential that you look at the listed programmes for your allocated deanery and consider your preferences before the selection centre to avoid any added stress on the day. While all programmes will have similar educational content, it is worth recognizing that some deaneries are large and therefore your decision on the programme may be influenced by geography. We recommend going to the selection centre with your mind made up, so you are not deliberating on these options when you should be focusing on getting through!

Deanery	Programmes	Website details
East of England	Basildon, Bedford, Bury St Edmunds, Cambridge, Chelmsford, Colchester, Great Yarmouth (Broadland), Harlow (West Essex), Hemel Hempstead and Watford, Huntingdon, Ipswich, Kings Lynn, Stevenage, Luton, Norwich, Peterborough, Southend, Welwyn Garden City	www.eoedeanery.nhs.uk
East Midlands	Boston, Chesterfield, Derby, Kettering, Leicester, Lincoln, Mansfield, Northampton, Nottingham, Worksop and Retford (North Notts)	www.eastmidlandsdeanery.nhs.uk
Kent, Surrey and Sussex	East Kent, West Kent, East Sussex, West Sussex, East Surrey, West Surrey	www.kssdeanery.org
London	North Central: Barnet, Enfield, UCLH, Bloomsbury and Royal Free, Whittington North West: St Mary's, Riverside, Central Middlesex, Northwick Park, West Middlesex, Hillingdon, Ealing North East: Romford, Hackney, Whipps Cross, Tower Hamlets, Newham, Ilford South West: St Helier, Kingston & Roehampton, Croydon, St Georges South East: Lewisham, Guy's and St Thomas, Kings, Bromley, Sidcup, Greenwich	www.londondeanery.ac.uk
Mersey	Macclesfield, Chester, Wirral, Whiston, Southport and Ormskirk, Liverpool, North Cheshire, South Cheshire	www.merseypostgradgp.nhs.uk
Northern	East Cumbria, Northumbria, Tees Valley, West Cumbria	www.northerndeanery.org
Northern Ireland	Northern Ireland	www.nimdta.gov.uk
Northwestern	South Academy: Bolton, Central Manchester, Pennine (North Manchester, Bury, Oldham and Rochdale), Salford and Trafford, South Manchester, Stockport, Tameside, Wigan North Academy: Blackpool, East Lancashire (Blackburn & Burnley), Lancaster, Ormskirk, Preston Chorley and District, South Cumbria	www.nwpgmd.nhs.uk

Deanery	Programmes	Website details
Oxford	Aylesbury, Wycombe, Banbury, Milton Keynes, Oxford, Reading and Newbury, Windsor	www.nesc.nhs.uk
Scotland	North of Scotland: Grampian, Highlands and Islands South East of Scotland: Borders and Midlothian, Fife and NE Edinburgh, West Lothian and West Edinburgh, Edinburgh and East Lothian, Central Edinburgh East of Scotland: Eastward, Westward West of Scotland: Ayrshire and Arran, Dumfries and Galloway, Glasgow North East, Glasgow North West, Glasgow South, Lanarkshire, Forth Valley, Renfrew, Inverslyde, Dumbarton and Argyll	www.nes.scot.nhs.uk/ medicine/continued_ practice/gp_careers
Severn	Gloucestershire, Swindon Cirencester, Bath, Bristol, Somerset	http://primarycare.severnd eanery.org
Southwest peninsula	Cornwall, Exeter, North Devon, Plymouth, Torbay	www.peninsuladeanery.nh s.uk
Wales	Aberystwyth, Bangor, Bridgend, Cardiff, Carmarthen, Dyffryn Clwyd, Glamorgan Valleys, Gwent, Neath Port Talbot, Pembrokeshire, Swansea, Wrexham	www.cardiff.ac.uk/pgmde/ sections/ general/specialty training/recr uitment
Wessex	Basingstoke, Bournemouth and Poole, Dorchester, Isle of Wight, Portsmouth, Salisbury, Southampton	www.nesc.nhs.uk
West Midlands	Coventry & Warwickshire, Shropshire, Stafford & Cannock, North Staffordshire & Keele University, Burton on Trent, Wolverhampton and Walsall, Dudley, East Birmingham/Solihull, North Birmingham, Sandwell & City, South Birmingham, North Worcestershire, South Worcester, Hereford	www.westmidlandsdeane ry.nhs.u k/GeneralPractice. aspx
Yorkshire and Humberside	North & East Yorkshire: Harrogate, Hull, Northallerton, North Lincolnshire, Scarborough, York South Yorkshire: Barnsley, Doncaster, Rotherham, Sheffield West Yorkshire: Airedale, Bradford, Dewsbury, Pontefract & Wakefield, Leeds, Pennine	www.yorksandhumberde anery.nh s.uk /general_pra ctice/applying/

SECTION C

Skills assessed by the GP ST entry process

4 The GP National Person Specification

Jasdeep Gill

Introduction

At each stage, your application and skills will be tested against the GPST National Person Specification which is an official document from the National Recruitment Office for General Practice. It is therefore important to familiarize yourself with this.

The GPST National Person Specification (NPS) outlines the competencies tested during the entry process and these will be broken down for you in this section. The specific sections in the book will refer back to the NPS to ensure you are familiar with it and appreciate how the NPS reflects the skills examiners are looking for during the GP entry process.

The NPS is divided into 'entry criteria' and 'selection criteria' with listed essential attributes which are discussed as we go along. The document also specifies in which part of the entry process the particular requirement will be tested. This should help you to understand the entry process and establish which particular skills are being tested at each stage.

Entry criteria

The entry criteria section of the NPS predominantly relates to stage 1 and looks at eight key areas:

1. Qualifications
2. Eligibility
3. Fitness to practise
4. Language skills
5. Health
6. Career progression
7. Application completion
8. Transportation.

Qualifications

This is an obvious one, but you must have a recognized primary medical qualification to apply. This can be MBBS or equivalent medical qualification and you will have to produce the original certificate when attending the stage 3 selection centre.

Eligibility

There are three key elements in assessing and demonstrating your eligibility. First, you must be eligible to work in the UK. Second, you must be fully registered with the UK General Medical Council (GMC) and hold a current licence to practise. For applicants who are required to take PLAB (Professional and Linguistic Assessment Board), you must have done so within 3 years of the potential commencement date of GP training for that year, or you must have progressed to clinical employment since taking PLAB.

Finally, you must have evidence of achievement of foundation competencies. If you are currently employed in a UK Foundation Programme Office (UKFPO)-affiliated Foundation Training Programme, then you will need to provide your FACD 5.2 (Foundation Achievement of Competence Document) once achieved. Alternatively, you will need to provide evidence of achievement of foundation competencies from a UKFPO-affiliated Foundation Programme or equivalent by the time of appointment, in line with GMC standards.

Fitness to practise

This is assessed by declaration in the application form and also on the structured reference form.

Language skills

You must have English language proficiency in both written and oral communication. These skills are required to a level which enables effective communication regarding medical topics with patients and colleagues. This requirement is practically tested at the stage 3 selection centre. However, in order to get to that stage you must have formal evidence of English language proficiency demonstrated in stage 1.

If you have undergone undergraduate medical training in English, then you do not need to produce any additional evidence, other than your original medical qualification certificate.

Alternatively, you will need to have achieved scores of 7 in a single sitting within 24 months of the time of application in the academic International English Language and Testing System (IELTS) in speaking, listening, reading, writing and overall.

If you believe that you have adequate communications skills, but do not have either of the above two requirements, then you must provide supporting evidence.

Health

You must meet the health requirements in line with the GMC standards. You must not put your patients at risk and must declare any condition which you could pass on to patients, or which could affect your judgement or performance.

This is assessed by declaration in stage 1, the structured reference form and also in the pre-employment health screening. All posts are subject to satisfactory pre-employment checks.

Career progression

The stage 1 application form will assess this aspect. You must not have any unexplained career gaps, nor have been released from or failed a GP specialty training programme or vocational training scheme previously, unless there are extraordinary circumstances.

Application completion

This should go without saying, but all applications must be fully completed and submitted before the deadline. No late submissions will be considered. Always bear in mind technical glitches with computer systems. It is essential to save your application as you go along and you should plan to submit it well in advance of the actual given deadline.

Transportation

This may seem a little odd to some, but for GP trainees transportation is essential. You require this to meet requirements of the whole training programme when providing emergency and domiciliary care. You will need to show evidence that you hold a current valid driving licence, or, agree to a statement of intent. Again, you will need to produce your original driving licence for verification at the stage 3 selection centre, or sign the statement of intent.

Selection criteria

The selection criteria form the bulk of the assessment in the GPST entry process. It is mainly assessed during stages 2 and 3, so it is imperative that you are familiar with it and appreciate how to demonstrate the essential skills. By understanding each requirement in the criteria, you will appreciate how to apply your skills in the GPST entry process and your daily practice.

This section will break down and explain each skill for you to ensure that you achieve a sound understanding of each requirement. We will revisit the criteria and outline the skills you should demonstrate for each part of the stage 3 selection centre in Chapters 11 and 12 with specific worked examples to help you apply the skills.

Selection criteria for GP ST National Person Specification

- Clinical skills
  - clinical knowledge and expertise
- Personal skills
  - empathy and sensitivity
  - communication skills
  - conceptual thinking and problem solving
  - coping with pressure
  - organization and planning
  - managing others and team involvement
- Probity
  - professional integrity
- Commitment to specialty
  - learning and personal development

Clinical knowledge and expertise

Capacity to apply sound clinical knowledge and awareness to full investigation of problems

GPST NPS statement

Your clinical skills and expertise will be assessed during the GPST entry process. As a doctor, you must be able to perform the following:

- be able to assimilate the data given to you;
- have a knowledge of aetiological factors and how to reduce risk;
- make correct diagnosis or differential diagnoses;
- have a knowledge of red flags;
- be able to order appropriate investigations;
- indicate first-line management plan;
- have a knowledge of common algorithms, including emergency care;
- consider follow up;

- have safe prescribing skills;
- have a knowledge of consent, confidentiality, refusal of investigation/treatment;
- have a correct management plan.

The vast majority of this skill set is assessed during the stage 2 assessment centre via the clinical problem-solving questions. Often the marks available for fulfilling this part of the NPS in stage 3 are relatively fewer: they are looking for the other key skills on that day. Nonetheless, you should aim to maximize your marks and we have given you some tips to help for each part of stage 3.

Empathy and sensitivity

Capacity and motivation to take in others' perspectives and to treat others with understanding.

GPST NPS statement

Doctors should have an understanding and sensitive manner. You can demonstrate empathy and sensitivity by exploring the situation from your patient's or colleague's perspective. Empathy and sensitivity includes the following:

- the patient as the central focus of care;
- treating others with respect, understanding and sensitivity;
- acknowledging the patient's problems and feelings;
- making others feel safe and be able to share their perspective.

You can carefully probe using open and closed questions to explore the patient's underlying concerns and expectations, which will help you gain an understanding of their perspective. For example, if breaking a new diagnosis, you should try to establish how this will impact on their life. You must not be judgemental or derogatory towards a patient or colleague.

Communication skills

Capacity to adjust behaviour and language as appropriate to the needs of differing situations.

GPST NPS statement

Communication skills are essential for every doctor. For GPs, effective communication is important due to time constraints on the length of consultations, the wide range of patients seen, the multitude of possible presentations of a given illness and the varying complexity of illness managed. Even though so much emphasis is placed on communication skills, some doctors sometimes struggle to communicate their thoughts or ideas effectively verbally or in writing. Reading hospital notes will demonstrate how much information is lost due to poor documentation – even if the individual writing the entry thought it made perfect sense. Therefore, the GPST entry process specifically assesses this skill in all three elements of the stage 3 selection centre.

Communication is a bidirectional process. You must convey your message with clarity using appropriate language, behaviour and non-verbal skills. It also requires you to listen, observe and be receptive to the communication from your patient or colleague. You must use jargon-free language and be able to adapt your style to suit the particular scenario. You may need to demonstrate that you can switch communication styles to adapt to new information, for example during stage 3. You will also need to demonstrate your skills in active listening and in absorbing information from patients and colleagues alike.

Conceptual thinking and problem solving

Capacity to think beyond the obvious, with an analytical and flexible mind.

GPST NPS statement

Your mind is your most powerful tool. Sometimes we have algorithms or protocols to follow which may help, but most often patients do not fit into neat boxes or follow the colourful arrows. What then? You have to think of a solution. As doctors, we need to use our clinical skills and judgement when problem solving, particularly when managing medical complexity and uncertainty.

Depending on the nature of the problem, there can be several possible approaches to solving it. The key steps involve identifying and clarifying the exact problem, analysing potential causes, thinking of options to solve the problem and then implementing a suitable option. Conceptual thinking is a helpful tool when problem solving. It relates to your ability to understand a problem by analysing patterns or connections and addressing the key underlying issues. It requires you to keep an open mind and think laterally or 'outside the box' when analysing the problem and thinking of solutions.

Coping with pressure

Capacity to recognize own limitations and develop appropriate coping mechanisms.
GPST NPS statement

Pressure and stress are intrinsic within the everyday role of doctors. It is well recognized that doctors have high levels of burnout, depression and even suicide. However, doctors often do not recognize symptoms in themselves. If using depression screening tools, 25% of GPs would be classed as suffering from depression. In essence, it is essential for all doctors to recognize such issues and have appropriate coping strategies for the safety of their patients and their own well-being.

Coping with pressure is a skill that can take years to hone. You are likely to have acquired some coping mechanisms during your training so far. Take a moment to think about your feelings when you are stressed and how you manage to cope with the pressure. Sometimes the most effective strategy is distancing yourself from your feelings and looking objectively at the situation and your response.

The first step to coping with pressure is being able to recognize it. Often several factors combine to cause high stress levels, but sometimes one factor affecting you continuously can be equally stressful. GPs often find the following factors cause increased stress levels:

- increased paperwork;
- insufficient time to manage patients in short consultation;
- increased demands from patients;
- increased demands and changes imposed by government/PCT;
- keeping up to date;
- job insecurity/self-employed status, financial concerns;
- feel isolated and difficult work–life balance;
- difficulty working with partners/colleagues;
- difficulties in running a practice as a viable business;
- employing and managing staff.

Knowing your limitations and recognizing stress early will help you implement coping strategies early. General approaches to coping with pressure include asking for help, organizing your time/workload efficiently, taking regular breaks (including planning and looking forward to annual leave), not taking on more work, have a social support network, talk about stresses openly (chances are everyone is going through similar stresses), see issues in context and not out of perspective.

Organization and planning

Capacity to organize information/time effectively in a planned manner.

GPST NPS statement

In both your professional and social lives, you organize and prioritize tasks every day. Sometimes you do it without even realizing. For example, if you still have to do your GPST application form and the deadline is tomorrow but your friends want to go out this evening, then you would automatically do your application form first and it is a no-brainer really – right?!

Other times it takes more conscious effort. For example, a scenario may be to prioritize a call back to a patient with indigestion or a call back to your babysitter who left a message on your voicemail sounding distressed. The patient with 'indigestion' may be having chest pain and you could assess this swiftly by taking a focused history by telephone and advising them to dial 999 if appropriate. However, there may be something wrong with your child or babysitter and you may not be able to focus until you know either way; but what if you have to rush off and what about the patient with indigestion? Consider which you would do first and why.

Time is often the key deciding factor when many people are organizing their tasks. However, as doctors, we have to remember that our actions (or lack of) could have serious consequences on patient safety and care.

Try using the prioritization matrix below to help you prioritize tasks. You should always attend to emergencies or urgent tasks immediately, whereas those which are not urgent or important can be attended to later.

	Urgent	Not urgent
Important	Emergencies Triaging telephone calls Some home visits Do it NOW!	Reviewing blood results Self-care (i.e. eat) Applications/exams Do it soon, could become 'urgent' if left too long
Not important	Some telephone calls Certain meetings Do it after urgent and important tasks	Chatting with colleague Reading a journal Do it once other tasks done

Managing others and team involvement

Capacity to work effectively in partnership with others
GPST NPS statement

Working as a team and individually while managing others is an essential part of general practice. Your skills to work effectively with others will be assessed in stage 3 and each exercise will require you to demonstrate this.

You should demonstrate that you can utilize the multidisciplinary team when managing chronic illness or that you can delegate tasks in the patient simulation and written prioritization exercise.

You should demonstrate your skills in supporting and motivating colleagues particularly in the group discussion. The key elements of managing others and team involvement to demonstrate include:

- awareness of each team member's roles;
- uses team members appropriately for patient care;
- delegates and negotiates appropriately with colleagues;
- awareness of personal and team actions on others;
- able to manage difficult colleagues;
- encouraging and supportive of colleagues.

Professional integrity

Capacity and motivation to take responsibility for own actions and demonstrate respect for all.

GPST NPS statement

The GMC Good Medical Practice guidelines highlight professional integrity and it forms an essential part of doctor's day-to-day duties. It is sometimes interchangeably referred to as 'probity.' The stage 2 professional dilemma questions will directly test your professional integrity and the stage 3 selection centre will require you to demonstrate this via your actions and comments. Use the list below to help apply your skills.

- Do not shirk responsibility.
- Take responsibility and be accountable for your actions.
- Be honest.
- Display mutual respect towards all.
- Appropriately disclose issues which may risk patient or public safety or your integrity.
- Act and operate within professional boundaries.
- Recognize your limitations.

Learning and personal development

Capacity and motivation to learn from experience and constantly update skills/knowledge.

GPST NPS statement

Lifelong learning and personal development are an important part of being a doctor. Opportunities for learning and development are endless and are around every corner in general practice. You should take charge of your learning and be motivated to identify your learning needs and address them.

Learning does not have to be done from a medical text book or by attending a course. You can learn vast amounts by reflecting on your daily clinical encounters and experiences. This skill is directly assessed in the stage 3 written prioritization exercise.

Use the pointers below to help you demonstrate your learning and personal development skills.

- Identify your learning needs.

- Reflect on and learn from your experiences.

- Show you can teach and learn through sharing with colleagues.

- Be motivated to learn new skills and information.

- Be supportive of others' learning needs and teaching opportunities.

- Maintain a portfolio and personal development plan.

- Be aware of lifelong learning, appraisal and revalidation.

As you work through the examples in this book, refer back to the summary of GP NPS regularly so that you understand the skills against which you are being assessed. You should also refer to the GMC Good Medical Practice guidelines and ensure that you fully understand the 'duties of a doctor' as you will find this helpful throughout the stage 3 selection centre and when answering the professional dilemma questions in stage 2. It will also prove very helpful to you throughout your career!

SECTION D

Stage 1: Application form

5 Registration and the on-line application

Jasdeep Gill

Introduction

Having decided that general practice is the career for you, you can proceed to the first stage of the GPST entry process: the application form. This chapter takes you through stage 1 and highlights the 'Dos and Don'ts' of the process.

Register

First things first, you will need to go through the registration process which will generate a personal record and specific applicant number for you. The application form is completed on-line via a link on the National GP Recruitment Office website. When registering your details, use an email address which you check regularly, because all communication will be done by email. Your email address will become your user-name within the application system.

Make sure you check your 'spam' folder in your email: important deanery emails sometimes get filtered as 'spam'. Don't get caught out and miss your invitation for the next stage!

Next you will have to confirm your deanery preferences. You can indicate a maximum of four deaneries in preference order. Your application form will undergo long-listing by your first choice deanery. You can change your deanery preferences and order once your application form has been submitted in case your circumstances change, but only within a stated time-frame. To complete your registration, you will need to enter your GMC number and confirm that you have a GMC valid licence to practise.

Application form

Once registered, you are ready to get going! However, before you get started, make sure you have the following information to hand:

- your primary medical degree and date of qualification;
- your employment history and a contact reference for each;
- the email address and details of three clinical referees;
- evidence of achievement of foundation competency or training, relevant certificates (i.e. for eligibility to work in the UK).

Most of the application form requires relatively factual and straightforward information. It has explanations for each section and uses mainly drop-down menus for you to select your response. You will not be asked any 'competency-based questions' nor have to give any lengthy essay-type answers.

There are several 'contextual questions' which evolve depending on the answer you select for the question before. You will require patience for these questions because it can be a little frustrating not knowing how many more questions are going to continue appearing on your screen! But bear with it and don't tear your hair out. Everybody has to go through the same process.

Make sure you complete and save each section as you go along. You do not have to finish and submit the form all in one sitting, but make sure you save your work regularly.

It is worth completing your application form well before the deadline: as with all computer-based systems, don't leave it to the last minute in case there is a 'server' or 'network' problem when everyone is trying to log on and complete it at the last minute.

Doing it on a reliable computer ideally at home is recommended. This helps avoid mistakes that will come from doing it on the ward during a lunch break!

The application form is lengthy with 10 sections to complete. We have noted the pertinent points for each section to help you crack through it.

Personal details section

When entering your address in this section bear in mind that it will be used to find the nearest available venue to you for the stage 2 assessment. Try to give the address of where you will be living at the time of the stage 2 assessment if you can. Alternatively, you can update your contact details on the system once you know.

Even though all the communication is done via email, always give a telephone number in case you need to be contacted urgently.

Foundation competency section

If you are currently employed on a UKFPO-affiliated foundation programme, then you simply need to give the name of your foundation school at this stage. Once you have achieved your foundation competencies and completed your foundation training, you will be awarded a FACD 5.2 certificate which you must submit to the deanery before a given deadline. Any offers made will be subject to you being awarded a FACD 5.2 certificate.

If you have already completed a UKFPO-affiliated foundation programme, simply give the name of your foundation school and either attach a copy of your FACD 5.2 certificate to your application form, or post a copy to your first choice deanery. You are advised not to do both because it could delay the processing of your application.

If you are in an alternative post or a stand-alone Foundation Year 2 post which is not affiliated with a foundation school, you will still need to provide evidence of foundation competency achievement.

Medicolegal section

You will need to confirm your status regarding transportation, medical defence insurance, occupational health and immigration. If you are an overseas doctor who can work in the UK without the need for a work permit, then your application will be considered alongside all other UK and EEA applicants. However, if you do require a work permit, your application will be considered, but an offer can only be made if there are no remaining suitable UK or EEA applicants.

Qualifications section

List your qualifications in reverse chronological order: your most recent qualification goes first. You will have to state a date, month and year. It is important to be accurate, but if you cannot remember the exact date, then enter '01/01/year' as a generic.

Within this section you should include additional qualifications and courses, particularly those which are relevant to GP training. This can be useful to demonstrate your commitment to specialty. For example, if you have done a diploma in a particular field relevant to general practice then clearly state this.

Experience section

List your previous jobs in reverse chronological order. Start with your current or most recent post and work backwards. For each post within a programme or year of training, you should add a separate entry. You must give full details of any career gaps longer than 4 weeks. Again you will have to state a date, month and year, and can use '01/01/year' if you cannot recall the exact date.

Reference section

Get the contact details of three clinical referees: your current supervisor, your last supervisor and the supervisor before that. You may have a choice of individual supervisors – if so, think carefully who will complete the forms reliably and on time.

 Bear in mind, a particular supervisor may be well renowned in your local area and therefore appear to be a 'star referee', but if they are too busy to complete the forms, you will do yourself a disservice.

It is courteous and appropriate to ask them beforehand, and when doing so, you can also confirm their preferred email, phone number and address. You should do this well in advance, so that you are able to enter their details straight into the application form without delay.

You are responsible for obtaining your three references. So you should download the 'structured reference form' from the GP National Recruitment Office website and send it to each referee as early as possible.

 Do it really early, in case they are away on leave later, busy or inundated with requests for other people's sign-offs and references – bear in mind this is often a busy time of year for everyone.

You will need to take all three of your complete reference forms to the stage 3 selection centre. You cannot proceed without them and this has been an unfortunate slip-up for candidates in the past.

Equal opportunities monitoring

This section is only used for monitoring purposes and has to be included by law, but does not form part of your application and you are not obliged to fill it in.

Fitness to practise and criminal conviction declaration

Be honest. If you have any previous fitness to practise enquiry or criminal conviction, then you must declare it. It may not necessarily prejudice your application.

Declaration

Read and 'sign' the declaration. Remember that an electronic signature is as valid as your signature on a paper-based application form.

Submit

Check through your application form very carefully and make sure all your changes have been saved. Once you have submitted your application form, you will be sent a confirmation email of receipt.

How to avoid having your application rejected at this stage

The application form itself is a relatively straightforward part of the entry process. However, you have to think about making yourself stand out from the crowd. Think about which audits or research to include and how you can demonstrate commitment to general practice. What additional work experience, if any, have you got under your belt? Consider which courses you have been on, or should now go on, to help demonstrate your desire to enter general practice. Your achievements can be valuable to display your commitment to general practice.

Obviously you will have to complete all the sections. Spelling errors and punctuation errors look sloppy and remember your web browser may not spellcheck your typing in the same manner as your word processor software. Some people prefer to type into a word processor and copy and paste into the boxes on the application form. This helps avoid spelling errors, but be sure to copy and paste the right sections into the right boxes!

Always ask someone to proofread your application and check for basic mistakes.

It is recommend that you use 'power' verbs when describing your achievements, for example, coordinated, directed, organized, negotiated, prioritized and established. Emphasize what you did and what you learnt and how it will help you for your career in general practice. Some applicants will have been involved in impressive research – however, you will not have done everything alone. The reviewers will want to know your individual involvement and what learning styles were used to gain from that experience. If you have done a lot of GP shadowing, demonstrate that you were active and not passively sitting in the corner. If you have done GP audits, then who came up with the question and how exactly did you collect the data. Did you complete the cycle and if not, why not?

Do not submit additional information or your curriculum vitae. It will not be considered or scored. It also shows you have not read the instructions properly.

If you have any career gaps of longer than 4 weeks, make sure you give full details of why and what you have done during this time. Apparently, employers could otherwise assume that you have been to prison – and we don't want that! In the past, career breaks were looked upon unfavourably. However, if you have done something interesting or exciting, then mention why you chose to do it and what you learnt. Make everything relevant to general practice: even diving in the Red Sea will involve learning new communication skills and working in a team.

Meet all deadlines and submit all the correct forms or certificates. Follow the instructions closely to avoid your application being delayed or rejected altogether.

Key points in completing the application form

- Read all instructions carefully.

- Only submit information that is asked for.

- Be honest with your answers.

- Be positive about all your experiences and relate them to general practice.

- Save your work at least every 10 minutes or it may get lost.

- Work on a familiar computer in a quiet place.

- Have patience with the 'contextual questions'.

- Submit your application form early, in case technical glitches occur.

- Late applications will not be considered.

SECTION E

Stage 2: Situational judgement assessment

Having made it over the first hurdle of stage 1, the deanery will invite you to stage 2 which consists of a situational judgement test (SJT). This section of the book will explain the format and outline the scoring for SJTs. It will prepare you for what to expect on the day to help ease your nerves and guide you on how to tackle the SJTs and highlight common themes which keep cropping up. The examples will help consolidate your understanding of the SJTs. You should use this section to help focus your revision and tackle those SJTs on the day.

6 Introduction to situational judgement tests

Jasdeep Gill

Use and format of the situational judgement test

The situational judgement test (SJT) is a form of psychometric testing which assesses your ability to apply your knowledge and skills in written scenarios. The questions are specifically written by GPs and the test is used to short-list applicants who score well and may be suitable for a career in general practice. The questions are carefully reviewed and validated to ensure they assess the required competencies based on the GP National Person Specification.

 Situational judgement tests were first used by US military psychologists during the Second World War.

The SJT is made up of two examination papers:

1. Clinical problem solving
2. Professional dilemmas.

The clinical problem-solving paper consists of clinical scenarios which test your problem solving, clinical judgement, diagnosis and management skills. It actually assesses your ability to apply your knowledge using clinical scenarios, rather than simply testing knowledge outright. The answer could relate to making a diagnosis, selecting an investigation, appropriate management, prescribing or emergency care. Some of the questions are 'best of five' and some are 'extending matching questions'.

The professional dilemmas paper uses clinical scenarios which encapsulate difficult situations with which a doctor could be presented. You will have to rank the responses in order of appropriateness. When reading the question, you should try to picture the patient or scenario and then answer the question. Think about the professional dilemma being posed and the skills being sort based on the National Person Specification. How would you apply those skills to solve the dilemma?

Both of the papers are pitched at a level suitable for Foundation Year 2 doctors and neither requires specific knowledge of general practice. However, the professional dilemmas paper may assume some awareness of common primary care areas, for example, in questions related to significant event analysis or gifts in primary care.

Scoring

Your score will determine whether or not you are short-listed. The scores for each paper are divided into four uneven sized 'bands' 1 to 4. The size of the bands and the score required to enter a band changes from year to year. This is because you are competing against your peers and the exam paper changes yearly. Band 1 is the lowest band and any applicant who scores within band 1 in one or both papers will not be short-listed. A breakdown of your results is emailed to you.

What to expect on the day

The stage 2 situational judgement assessment is traditionally a paper-based examination. However, the GP National Recruitment Office wants to computerize this assessment, potentially with effect from 2011. A computer-based assessment will allow applicants to visit a nearby 'Pearson Vue' test centre within a given window of time to sit an electronic version of the stage 2 assessment. You may have encountered computer-based assessments and Pearson Vue when you did your driving test. This section will give you an overview of the assessment at a Pearson Vue centre.

Register and select a suitable venue, date and time for your stage 2 assessment. You will need to take a proof of photographic identification with you, such as your driving licence or passport. You will not be allowed to take any food, drink, watches, calculators or personal items into the examination room with you, but you will be given a locker in which to leave everything. Make sure you don't arrive hungry!

Once you are seated at your computer terminal, you will go through key instructions on your computer. These will help familiarize you with how to click through the questions, how to select your answers, how to drag and drop your answers to the ranking questions, how to flag a question to review later and how to review your paper at the end. This will last approximately 10 minutes and it is important that you read through and follow these instructions to make sure you do not get confused or panic later.

A timer will count down in the top right of your screen. Remember that time will be tight, so keep an eye on the timer. Set yourself checkpoints, for example, check that you are at least a quarter of the way through the questions, once a quarter of the allocated time has elapsed. Do the same at half way through and again at three-quarters through. The assessment is not negatively marked, so do not leave any questions unanswered. If you do not know an answer, take an educated guess and flag it for review so that you can come back to it at the end. Do not dwell on any question for too long – the clock will continue ticking!

It is worthwhile looking away from the screen briefly every 20–30 minutes to help prevent your eyes becoming strained. There are no scheduled breaks during the examination. Unlike other written exams you have sat, you cannot take snacks or drinks. So go well fed and hydrated, but factor in taking a toilet break into your timing. Both papers for the stage 2 assessment may run one directly after the other.

7 Insider's guide to answering SJT questions

Jasdeep Gill

Introduction

Best of five questions

For the best of five questions, you are given a clinical scenario and then following statements, which may be 'diagnoses', 'tests' or any number of things. You must select the single best statement that best answers the question. Remember to read the question carefully. For example, while many say 'what is the right statement?', there are some which are negatively phrased and say 'which is not the next step?'.

Be wary of selecting the first 'best' statement as you read the options: read all the statements and then eliminate the statements which are clearly wrong. You can usually eliminate two options as wrong, with another being eliminated by applying logic. Therefore, you have rapidly got a choice of two. Hopefully, you will know the answer. If you don't, then don't panic, and go with your instincts. Some people find that their 'instinct stinks'! You can improve your instincts by practising questions, studying the explanations for the answers and by reviewing a brief medical text book. You should not try to digest a large tome, it will only panic you and theoretically you should already have the knowledge and skills to pass this test.

Extended matching questions

For extended matching questions, you are given several different statements or potential answers. The question is often in the form of a clinical scenario. You must match the statements to the scenarios. Again, read all the options carefully and check all the words – a statement may appear to be 'correct', but have a caveat. For example, when considering INR ranges for a first pulmonary embolism, an option may include 'INR 2–3 for 3 months' and 'INR 2–3 for 6 months'. Your eye may spot the '2–3' part of the statement in amongst a list of inappropriate INR ranges, but watch out for the qualifying time. In this example, the latter option is correct.

Professional dilemmas

In the professional dilemma questions, it really pays to put yourself in the shoes of the individual in the scenario. It is possible that you have actually experienced a similar event occurring in your hospital. However, it is better to think what should be done, rather than what actually happened in your experience. These questions take a great deal more thought than the clinical problem solving and you must 'get in the head' of the examiner. In reality, this is not as hard as it sounds because all the questions will be based around key parts of the person specification and the key GMC documents – 'Duties of a doctor' and 'Good medical practice'. Always prioritize patient safety, never collude with illegal activities and aim to tackle the situation at hand rather than deferring it or 'passing the buck' to another individual. Always apply logic and think of what steps you would take to sort out the dilemma. While some people will tell you that you cannot revise for these questions, you can certainly improve your technique and approach by practise.

Top tip

- Answer ALL the questions:
    - There is no negative marking, so take an educated guess if you have to.
- Time is of the essence!
    - Do NOT procrastinate over a particular question for long.
    - If you don't know, make a definite decision based on your instincts.
    - Mark your answer and move on.
- Have energy bars or some long-lasting complex carbohydrates before the exam.
- Put yourself in the shoes of the individuals in the scenario.
- Draw upon your clinical experience: have you seen this happen before? If so, what did you do? What should you have done if that didn't go well?

Questions can have terminology that is essential to answer correctly. Beware of:

Pathognomic/diagnostic/characteristic: >90% of cases	For example, Koplick spots in measles Not to have this clinical feature would place the diagnosis in doubt
Typical/common/significant/frequent: >60% of cases	For example, pericardial friction rub in pericarditis This feature will help you diagnose the condition but is not always present
Minority: <50% of cases	
Majority: >50% of cases	
Low chance: <30% of cases	
Recognized/reported: not related to frequency	For example, it is recognized that aortic root dilation occurs in ankylosing spondylitis

Common themes for the SJT

The clinical problem-solving questions will include questions from medicine, surgery, therapeutics and several specialties.

Within your revision, you should aim to cover a wide range of areas and topics.

 Use the table to do an initial self-rating assessment of your knowledge in all the areas. This should help you identify your weaknesses and focus your revision.

	Insufficient knowledge	Need further development	Competent
Cardiovascular			
Dermatology			
ENT			
Ophthalmology			
Gastroenterology			
Infectious disease			
Haematology			
Immunology			
Genetics			
Musculoskeletal			
Paediatrics			
Pharmacology			
Neurology			
Reproductive (female and male)			
Renal			
Respiratory			
Urology			

It is really tempting to relearn areas which you already know, because the familiarity of it and doing it well is comforting. Avoid this temptation! You should identify your learning needs and focus your learning according to that. Edit the table as you progress with your revision. Hopefully you will feel confident and have the 'competent' box ticked for all the areas prior to the exam.

8 Clinical problem solving: questions and answers

Rajesh Kumar and Sukhjinder Nijjer

Questions

Cardiovascular: *Multiple Choice Questions*

1. A 55-year-old male presents to morning surgery with a history of exertional chest pain. He is a known diabetic on insulin. A recent blood test showed elevated HDL (high-density lipoprotein) and he admits to smoking 20 cigarettes per day. Which of the following is not associated with coronary artery disease?
    - A. Male gender
    - B. Increased HDL
    - C. Hypertension
    - D. Diabetes
    - E. Cigarette smoking

2. A 55-year-old male is admitted to hospital with chest pain and has a STEMI (ST segment elevation myocardial infarction). He underwent a primary percutaneous coronary intervention (PCI). He is discharged from hospital and on the same day has come to see you in general practice. He would like to return to work immediately as a HGV driver. When can he return to work (select one option)?
    - A. Immediately
    - B. After 1 week
    - C. After 2 weeks
    - D. After 4 weeks
    - E. After at least 6 weeks.

3. An 87-year-old man is rushed into A&E resus by ambulance having collapsed at home after complaining of chest pain. The paramedics are on the third cycle of cardiopulmonary resuscitation (CPR). The rhythm is checked and shows pulseless electrical activity (PEA). Which one of the following should be done next?

    A. Deliver one shock and immediately resume CPR at 30:2

    B. Immediately resume CPR at 30:2

    C. Deliver one shock and give adrenaline

    D. Immediately resume CPR at 15:2

    E. Deliver one shock and immediately resume CPR at 15:2.

4. Which of the following is not a feature seen on chest x-ray of a person with left ventricular failure? (select one option only):

    A. Pleural effusion

    B. Kerley Z lines

    C. Alveolar oedema

    D. Upper lobe blood diversion

    E. Cardiomegaly.

5. A 65-year-old female presents in the early hours of the morning with acute dyspnoea and pink frothy sputum. You note that she is sitting up, very distressed, pale, sweating and has an elevated JVP (jugular venous pressure). Which is the single most likely cause for her symptoms? (select one option only):

    A. Chronic obstructive pulmonary disease (COPD)

    B. Pneumonia

    C. Pulmonary oedema

    D. Small pleural effusion

    E. Anxiety.

Cardiovascular: *Extended Matching Questions*

For each of the following scenarios, choose the most appropriate management from the options below (each option may be selected once, more than once or not at all):

    A. Warfarin with INR 2.5 for 3 months
    B. Warfarin with INR 3.5 for 3 months
    C. Warfarin with INR 4.0 for 3 months
    D. Warfarin with INR 2.5 for 6 months
    E. Warfarin with INR 3.5 for 6 months
    F. Warfarin with INR 4.0 for 6 months
    G. Lifelong warfarin
    H. No anticoagulation required
    I. None of the above.

6. A 42-year-old man diagnosed with a proximal DVT and no risk factors.

7. A 60-year-old obese woman with a newly diagnosed PE.

8. A 32-year-old pregnant woman with DVT.

For each of the following scenarios, choose the most appropriate management from the options below (each option may be selected once, more than once or not at all):

    A. Investigate for underlying cause
    B. Urgent treatment and referral needed
    C. Start on ramipril
    D. Reassess in 5 years
    E. Start on bisoprolol
    F. Reassess annually
    G. Start on amlodipine
    H. Start on bendrofluthiazide
    I. Do nothing.

9. A 30-year-old man with a family history of late-onset diabetes has a blood pressure of 158/74.

10. A 55-year-old woman on ramipril and amlodipine recently stopped her medications since returning from holiday. She comes for a routine appointment with the practice nurse for a blood pressure (BP) check. Her BP reading is 225/120. She feels systemically well.

11. A 63-year-old Afro-Caribbean man has a blood pressure of 134/86

For each of the following scenarios, choose from the diagnoses below (each option may be selected once, more than once or not at all):

    A. Pulmonary embolism
    B. Decubitus angina
    C. Unstable angina
    D. Myocardial infarction
    E. Dissecting aortic aneurysm
    F. Acute pericarditis
    G. Ruptured abdominal aortic aneurysm (AAA).

12. A 35-year-old male who has used large amounts of cocaine at a party presents to A&E with crushing central chest pain and clamminess.

13. A 65-year-old women experiences exertional chest pain relieved by GTN. More recently, she has noticed that her chest pain is precipitated by lying flat.

14. A 35-year-old male has sharp central chest pain that is worse with inspiration and relieved sitting forwards.

Dermatology/ENT/Eye: *Multiple Choice Questions*

1. A 75-year-old male has noticed a bleeding lesion on the side of his nose. You notice a small pearly-white nodule with visible blood vessels. Which is the single most likely cause for his symptoms? (select one option only):

    A. Actinic keratoses
    B. Rat ulcer
    C. Basal cell carcinoma
    D. Malignant melanoma
    E. Bowen's disease.

2. A 3-year-old boy attends the surgery with his mother who states that he has been generally unwell with a temperature for the past 3 days. He has also been tugging and complaining that his left ear hurts. On examination, there is a hyperaemic bulging left ear drum. Which is the single most likely cause for his symptoms? (select one option only):

    A. Acute otitis externa
    B. Cholesteatoma
    C. Acute otitis media

D. Otosclerosis

E. Mastoiditis.

3. A 40-year-old male with nasal obstruction has been diagnosed with bilateral nasal polyps. He suffers seasonal hay fever, but is otherwise well. Which of the following is not associated with nasal polyps? (select one option only):

A. Allergic rhinitis

B. Aspirin sensitivity

C. Chronic ethmoidal sinusitis

D. Cystic fibrosis

E. Eczema.

4. A 24-year-old colour-blind man requests a medical check as part of his application to be a taxi driver. He is fit and well. What should you advise him regarding DVLA notification and his colour blindness? (select one option only):

A. To inform the DVLA and stop driving

B. To inform the DVLA and can drive

C. Not to inform the DVLA

D. Not to inform the DVLA and can drive

E. Not to inform the DVLA and stop driving.

5. Which of the following is not a feature of hypertensive retinopathy? (select one option only):

A. Silver wiring

B. Papilloedema

C. Cotton wool spots

D. AV nipping

E. None of the above.

6. A 16-year-old type 1 diabetic enquires about how often she should be having screening for diabetic retinopathy. For the options below, select the most appropriate response (select one option only):

A. None at present because too young to have changes

B. Once every 6 months

C. Once every year

D. Once every 2 years

E. If she notices any visual change.

7. A 16-year-old male complains of an acute onset of bilateral gritty and discharging eyes. His vision is normal. On examination, there is marked crusting of the eyelid margin with conjunctival injection. Which two options are appropriate in his management? (select two options only):

    A. Do nothing
    B. Refer to A&E
    C. Eyelid hygiene
    D. Topical chloramphenicol
    E. Oral metronidazole.

Dermatology/ENT/eye: *Extended Matching Questions*

For each of the following scenarios, choose from the diagnoses below (each option may be selected once, more than once or not at all):

    A. Psoriasis
    B. Atopic eczema
    C. Impetigo
    D. Cellulitis
    E. Trigeminal zoster
    F. Tinea pedis
    G. Intertrigo.

8. A mother is concerned about her 1-year-old daughter who has a rash on her face, neck and limbs. There is marked redness over the face with scaling and evidence of scratching. The skin is very dry with widespread blotchy erythema, including the antecubital and popliteal fossae.

9. A 72-year-old female presents with a vesicular rash involving the left side of her face, including the left side of her nose. The rash was preceded by pain.

10. A 55-year-old male with a body mass index (BMI) of 40 presents with wet maceration to the skin in the submammary region.

For each of the following scenarios, choose from the diagnoses below (each option may be selected once, more than once or not at all):

    A. Polymorphic eruption of pregnancy
    B. Pruritus gravidarum
    C. Exacerbation eczema
    D. Pemphigoid gestationis
    E. Varicella zoster
    F. Exacerbation psoriasis
    G. Impetigo herpetitformis
    H. Allergic reaction.

11. A 34-year-old pregnant woman in the third trimester complains of extremely itching palms and soles, so much so that she has caused excoriations from scratching. You note that she has abnormal liver function tests.

12. A 26-year-old primiparous woman presents in the third trimester with extremely itchy abdominal striae and small urticarial lesions extending on her thighs. On examination, you note periumbilical sparing.

13. A 32-year-old Asian woman presents to you with a localized rash on her back since the morning. She is 26 weeks pregnant and does not know her immunization status.

For each of the following scenarios, choose from the diagnoses below (each option may be selected once, more than once or not at all):

    A. Measles
    B. Mumps
    C. Rubella
    D. Meningococcal septicaemia
    E. Herpes zoster
    F. Polio
    G. Tuberculosis.

14. A 4-year-old boy with a fever and coryza for 4 days develops an erythematous maculopapular rash. He also has tiny white spots on the buccal mucosa of the cheeks.

15. A 2-year-old girl develops a pink macular rash behind her ears and on her face. Over the course of 4 days, this spreads to the trunk and spontaneously resolves. There is some mild cervical lymphadenopathy.

16. A 5-year-old boy looks unwell with a temperature of 38.2°C. His mother tells you that she has noticed a non-blanching rash.

For each of the following scenarios, choose from the above diagnoses (each option may be selected once, more than once or not at all):

    A. Barotrauma
    B. Wax/foreign body
    C. Otitis media with effusion
    D. Acoustic neuroma
    E. Menière's disease
    F. Drug induced
    G. Presbyacusis.

17. A 22-year-old male has recently returned from a long-haul flight from Australia. He reports marked pain in his right ear along with hearing loss.

18. A 55-year-old female has noticed episodic attacks of dizziness and ringing in her ears. During each attack, her hearing is significantly reduced.

19. A 70-year-old female has noticed that it is becoming increasingly difficult to have a conversation in a crowded room. She can manage one-to-one conversation in a quiet room.

For each of the following scenarios, choose the most suitable management option from the list below (each option may be selected once, more than once or not at all):

    A. Watchful waiting
    B. Antibiotic treatment
    C. Monospot testing
    D. HIV testing
    E. Referral for intravenous antibiotics
    F. Referral for bronchoscopy
    G. None of the above.

20. A 16-year-old female developed a sore throat 3 months previously with cervical lymphadenopathy. She reports that she is tired all of the time.

21. A 16-year-old female has had unresolving tonsillitis for the past 2 weeks. She has now developed earache, severe dysphagia and difficulty opening her mouth.

22. A 32-year-old male returns from a business trip to Thailand 6 weeks previously. He reports feeling generally unwell with fever and sore throat. He admits to unprotected intercourse.

For each of the following scenarios, choose from the diagnoses below (each option may be selected once, more than once or not at all):

    A. Subconjuctival haemorrhage
    B. Keratitis
    C. Acute glaucoma
    D. Anterior uveitis
    E. Episcleritis
    F. Central retinal artery occlusion
    G. Conjunctivitis
    H. Hypopyon
    I. Central retinal vein occlusion
    J. Corneal ulceration
    K. Scleritis.

23. A 65-year-old woman presents with a painful left red eye and reduced visual acuity. She has associated nausea and vomiting. Examination reveals a fixed semi-oval pupil, periocular pain and congestion.

24. A 27-year-old man with Bcchet's disease presents with a congested right eye. He reports using steroid eye drops recently for a sore red eye. Examination reveals a yellowish fluid level in the anterior chamber.

25. An 87-year-old hypertensive man reports a sudden painless loss of vision in his left eye. Examination reveals a pale retina and 'cherry red spot'.

Endocrinology/metabolic medicine: *Multiple Choice Questions*

1. A female patient thinks that she has diabetes, as she has been getting very thirsty and passing frequent amounts of urine. What random venous glucose level would confirm diagnosis? (select one option only):

   A. >6.6
   B. >7
   C. <10.5
   D. ≥11.1
   E. None of the above.

2. A 45-year-old lady attends surgery and has a BMI of 29. She is diagnosed as having type 2 diabetes mellitus that is not controlled despite her best efforts at lifestyle change. What would be the next step in her management? (select one option only):

   A. Do nothing
   B. Start a biguanide
   C. Start a sulfonylurea
   D. Commence insulin
   E. Refer her for bariatric surgery.

3. Which of the following hormones is released from the posterior pituitary gland? (select one option only):

   A. Prolactin
   B. Oxytocin
   C. Thyroid stimulating hormone
   D. Growth hormone
   E. Luteinizing hormone.

4. Which of the following is associated with a reduced risk of developing type 2 diabetes? (select one option only):

   A. Asian ethnicity
   B. History of diabetes in parents
   C. History of pregnancy-induced diabetes
   D. Exercise
   E. Obesity.

Endocrinology/metabolic medicine: *Extended Matching Items*

For each of the following scenarios, choose from the diagnoses below (each option may be selected once, more than once or not at all):

    A. Addison's disease
    B. Menopause
    C. Conn's syndrome
    D. Diabetes insipidus
    E. Depression
    F. Diabetes mellitus
    G. Mendleson's syndrome
    H. Sheehan's syndrome
    I. Phaeochromocytoma
    J. Cushing syndrome.

5. A 34-year-old woman who recently suffered post-partum haemorrhage reports difficulty breastfeeding, fatigue, lack of energy and failure to resume her menstruation.

6. A 53-year-old lady reports that when she gets stressed she suffers with a combination of panic attacks and can feel her heart racing away. She has high blood pressure.

7. A 50-year-old female is on long-term prednisolone for arthritis. She has noticed significant weight gain, lethargy, irritability, excessive facial hair and purple stretch marks on her abdomen.

For each of the following scenarios, choose the most appropriate medication from the list below (each option may be selected once, more than once or not at all). Normal ranges: FSH 0.8–11.5 U/L, LH 0.8–12 U/L, T4 8–22 pmol/L and TSH 0.35–5.5 mIU/L.

    A. Carbimazole
    B. Carbimazepine
    C. Clonidine
    D. Clotrimazole
    E. Metformin
    F. Azithromycin

G. Azothioprine
H. Metoprolol
I. Propylthiouracil
J. Fluoxetine
K. Levothyroxine
L. Co-carledopa
M. HRT
N. Amitripyline.

8. A 42-year-old woman presents with menorrhagia, low mood and weight gain. Her blood test reveal: Hb 12.1 g/L, Platelets 288 × 109/L, TSH 16 mIU/L, 3 pmol/L, FSH 8 U/L.

9. A 33-year-old pregnant woman, who is normally fit and well, presents with palpitations and heat intolerance. Her blood tests reveal Hb 11.2, platelets 350 × 109/L, TSH 0.2 mIU/L, free T4 24 pmol/L and FSH 9.5 U/L.

10. A 22-year-old overweight woman presents with subfertility. Her current partner has one child and she has none. Her blood tests reveal Hb 11.8 g/L, platelets 290 × 109/L, TSH 4 mIU/L, free T4 12 pmol/L, LH 14 U/L and FSH 4.2 U/L. Ultrasound revealed cysts in the ovaries, but other investigations, including hysterosalpingogram, were normal.

Gastroenterology/nutrition: *Multiple Choice Questions*

1. A 56-year-old man presents with a 3-month history of intractable dyspepsia and generalized weight loss. Which one of the following is the most appropriate management? (select one option only):
    A. Urgent referral for colonoscopy
    B. Urgent referral for oesophago-gastro-duodenoscopy
    C. Urgent referral for cytoscopy
    D. Urgent referral for bronchoscopy
    E. Reassure.

Gastroenterology/nutrition: *Extended Matching Questions*

For each of the following scenarios, choose from the diagnoses in the list below (each option may be selected once, more than once or not at all):

    A. Ulcerative colitis
    B. Gastro-oesophageal reflux disease (GORD)
    C. Irritable bowel syndrome (IBS)
    D. Primary biliary cirrhosis (PBC)
    E. Coeliac disease
    F. Autoimmune hepatitis (AIH).

2. A 19-year-old female attends with central abdominal pain (relieved by defaecation), abdominal bloating and altered bowel habit. She states that she has been under a lot of work-related stress for the past 6 months and her bowel symptoms started at a similar time.

3. A 25-year-old male presents with a gradual onset of diarrhoea with both blood and mucus mixed with the stool. He has associated cramping abdominal discomfort.

4. A 50-year-old female with a background of rheumatoid arthritis presents with an 8-month history of lethargy and pruritis. She reports that her family think she looks yellow.

For each of the following scenarios below, choose from the most appropriate tumour marker to help distinguish the diagnosis (each option may be selected once, more than once or not at all):

    A. Carcinoembryonic antigen
    B. Alpha-feto protein
    C. Bence–Jones protein
    D. Prostate-specific antigen
    E. Calcitonin
    F. TSH
    G. CA 19–9
    H. CA 15–3
    I. CA 125
    J. Gamma glutamyl transferase
    K. Liver alkaline phosphatase
    L. Bone alkaline phosphatase.

5. An 84-year-old man presents with back pain, lethargy and urinary hesitancy. He recently had a fall while getting up in the night to pass urine. He has experienced gradual generalized weight loss.

6. A 38-year-old man presents with a unilateral neck lump, intractable facial flushing and diarrhoea. He reports a familial predisposition to tumours.

7. An 82-year-old nulliparous woman presents with lower abdominal discomfort and bloating, but generalized weight loss.

For each of the following scenarios, choose your most appropriate action (each option may be selected once, more than once or not at all):

A.   Urine dipstick
B.   Bence–Jones protein
C.   Routine referral to medical team
D.   Routine referral to surgical team
E.   Chest x-ray
F.   Abdominal ultrasound
G.   Give laxatives
H.   Give zopiclone
I.   Reassure
J.   Urgent referral to medical team
K.   Urgent referral to surgical team.

8. A 69-year-old woman with abdominal pain, nausea and vomiting. The nurses inform you that she has not opened her bowels for 5 days. You note a tender distended abdomen and tympanic bowel sounds.

9. A 19-year-old law student presents complaining of constipation with nausea and lower abdominal discomfort. She reports being stressed with exams and amenorrhoea. She would like something to solve the constipation and help her sleep.

10. A 24-year-old anxious man presents after painful defaecation and having noticed a small amount of bright red blood on wiping. He is well with no constitutional or concerning symptoms.

Infectious disease/haematology/immunology/genetics:
Multiple Choice Questions

1. A 19-year-old female is diagnosed as having chlamydia during antenatal testing. Which one of the following is the most appropriate treatment? (select one option only):
    - A. Doxycycline
    - B. Azithromycin
    - C. Erythromycin
    - D. Metronidazole
    - E. Penicillin V.

2. On a routine blood test, a patient is shown to have a low haemoglobin with a MCV (mean corpuscular volume) of 100 fL. Which of the following is not a cause of a macrocytic anaemia? (select one option only):
    - A. B12 deficiency
    - B. Folate deficiency
    - C. Iron deficiency
    - D. Cytotoxic drug use
    - E. Excess alcohol.

3. A 40-year-old pregnant female attends during afternoon surgery concerned that she may be at increased risk of having a baby with Down syndrome. She is due to have her 11-week ultrasound scan. Which of the following increase the likelihood of Down's syndrome? (select one option):
    - A. High maternal age
    - B. Gender of fetus
    - C. Reduced nuchal translucency on ultrasound
    - D. Low human chorionic gonadotrophin beta subunit
    - E. Excess maternal exercise.

4. A 25-year-old cleaner who is 5 weeks pregnant enquires about folic acid supplements. She is healthy, with no past medical history. Which of the following is correct? (select one option only):
    - A. 4 mg daily
    - B. 400 µg daily
    - C. 0.4 µg daily
    - D. 5 mg daily
    - E. None, because she is healthy and already pregnant.

5. Which of the following vaccines are live? (select two options):
   A. Rubella
   B. Tetanus
   C. BCG
   D. Pertussis
   E. Flu jab.

6. Which congenital infection would be the most likely cause of a stillbirth with hydrops fetalis, which was rhesus-compatible? (select one option only):
   A. Toxoplasmosis
   B. Parvovirus
   C. Rubella
   D. Cytomegalovirus
   E. Herpes simplex virus.

7. What is the mode of inheritance for cystic fibrosis? (select one option only):
   A. Autosomal dominant
   B. Autosomal recessive
   C. X-linked dominant
   D. X-linked recessive
   E. Multifactorial.

8. A 10-year-old boy is stung by a wasp. He develops anaphylaxis and is rushed to hospital. What dose of adrenaline should he be given? (select one option only):
   A. 500 µg intramuscular of 1:1 000 adrenaline
   B. 500 µg intramuscular of 1:10 000 adrenaline
   C. 300 µg intramuscular of 1:1000 adrenaline
   D. 300 µg intramuscular of 1:10 000 adrenaline
   E. 150 µg intramuscular of 1:10 000 adrenaline.

9. A 31-year-old haemophilia carrier asks you about the chances of her having an affected child, with her unaffected husband. Which of the following is false? (select one option only):
   A. No risk of the father passing it to his sons
   B. 1 in 2 risk of having a carrier daughter
   C. 1 in 2 risk of having an affected son

    D. 1 in 4 risk of having an affected child

    E. 1 in 4 risk of having an affected son.

10. What is the term used to describe the phenomenon where the signs and symptoms of a genetic condition appears earlier and is more severe in successive generations? (select one option only):

    A. Lyonization

    B. Anticipation

    C. Translocation

    D. Ageism

    E. Amplification.

11. Which of the following are not notifiable diseases? (select three options):

    A. Meningitis

    B. Chicken pox

    C. Salmonella

    D. Tuberculosis

    E. Infectious mononucleosis

    F. Scarlet fever

    G. Pertussis

    H. Leprosy

    I. Anthrax

    J. Schistosomiasis

    K. Cholera

    L. Enchephalitis.

Infectious disease/haematology/immunology/genetics: *Extended Matching Questions*

For each of the following scenarios, choose your most appropriate diagnosis from the list below (each option may be selected once, more than once or not at all):

    A. Chlamydia

    B. Gonorrhoea

    C. Candida

    D. Scabies

    E. Genital warts

    F. HPV

G. Bacterial vaginosis
H. Trichomonas vaginalis
I. HIV
J. Syphillis.

12. A 28-year-old teacher presents with a 2-week history of offensive thin vaginal discharge, particularly after sexual intercourse. She reports cleaning herself meticulously to help, but it will not go away.

13. A 28-year-old librarian presents with thick creamy vaginal discharge and vulvovaginal itching, particularly worse premenstrually and at night.

14. A 28-year-old accountant presents with offensive thin vaginal discharge which she describes as 'greeny and frothy'.

For each of the following scenarios, choose your most appropriate diagnosis (each option may be selected once, more than once or not at all):

A. Thalassaemia
B. Sickle cell disease
C. Pernicious anaemia
D. Iron deficiency anaemia
E. Anaemia of chronic disease
F. Sideroblastic anaemia
G. Aplastic anaemia
H. Folate deficiency
I. Alcoholism
J. Haemolytic anaemia.

15. A 62-year-old woman with vitiligo presents with lethargy and feeling tired all the time. She reports going through premature menopause and had premature greying of her hair. Blood test reveal: Hb 8.9 g/L, MCV 106 fL.

16. A 67-year-old man complains of feeling tired all the time. He has recently suffered with recurrent bacterial infections. He has recently noted that his gums bleed for no apparent reason and he has developed widespread unexplained bruising. Blood tests reveal:

Hb 10.1 g/L, MCV 92 fL, platelets 20×109/L, blood film shows hypocellularity.

17. A 56-year-old post-menopausal woman complains of feeling tired all the time. She has noticed difficulty in swallowing and has become pale. She is also concerned that her tongue feels sore and her nails have become 'dipped in like a spoon'. Blood tests reveal: Hb 9.5 g/L, MCV 78 fL, blood film poikilocytes.

For each of the following scenarios, choose the most likely chromosomal configuration (each option may be selected once, more than once or not at all):

    A. 46 XO
    B. 45 XO
    C. 46 XXY
    D. Trisomy 21
    E. 46 XX
    F. 47 XXX
    G. 47 XXY
    H. Trisomy 18
    I. 46 XY
    J. Trisomy 13
    K. 46 XXX.

18. A short 15-year-old girl with widely spaced nipples but absent secondary sexual characteristics.

19. A tall 22-year-old man presents with infertility. Examination reveals gynaecomastia, but otherwise normal masculinization.

20. An 8-month-old baby with low set ears, micrognathia and rocker-bottom feet.

Musculoskeletal: *Multiple Choice Questions*

1. A 72-year-old woman was walking to the GP practice and slipped on the ice falling onto an outstretched left hand. She noticed immediate pain and swelling. On examination of the left wrist there is marked swelling, bruising with deformity. What is the likely diagnosis? (select one option only):
   A. Smith's fracture
   B. Barton's fracture
   C. Colles' fracture
   D. Bennett's fracture-dislocation
   E. Jones' fracture.

Musculoskeletal: *Extended Matching Questions*

For each of the following scenarios, choose your most appropriate diagnosis (each option may be selected once, more than once or not at all):

   A. Ankylosing spondylitis
   B. Leaking abdominal aortic aneurysm
   C. Mechanical back pain
   D. Sciatica
   E. Osteoporosis
   F. Primary neoplasm
   G. Cauda equina syndrome
   H. Polymyalgia rheumatica
   I. Myeloma.

2. A 66-year-old male presents with a history of lethargy, weight loss and lower back pain. Recent blood tests show that he is anaemic and has renal impairment.

3. A 35-year-old female has lower back pain with radiation down both legs. She has noted significant lower leg weakness and is now having unnoticed leakage of urine.

4. A 60-year-old female has stiffness around the shoulder and pelvic girdle. She has intermittent lower back pain. Over the past few days she had been experiencing malaise.

For each of the following scenarios, choose your most appropriate diagnosis (each option may be selected once, more than once or not at all):

    A. Juvenile onset arthritis
    B. Gout
    C. Osteoarthritis
    D. Rheumatoid arthritis
    E. Septic arthritis
    F. Psoriatic arthritis
    G. Pyogenic arthritis
    H. Pseudogout.

5. A 50-year-old female reports progressive pain in her right knee over the past 2 months. The pain is exacerbated by walking and relieved with rest. She has early morning stiffness.

6. A 6-year-old boy has a red, painful and swollen left knee, held in a slightly flexed position. He has no history of trauma. His mother reports that he had a temperature of 38.5° during the night.

7. A 70-year-old male has a sudden onset of right knee pain and swelling. A sample of synovial fluid shows positively birefringent crystals.

For each of the following scenarios, choose your most appropriate diagnosis (each option may be selected once, more than once or not at all):

    A. Bursitis
    B. Congenital dislocation of the hip (CDH)
    C. Juvenile onset arthritis
    D. Perthes' disease
    E. Slipped upper femoral epiphysis (SUFE)
    F. Septic arthritis
    G. Transient synovitis
    H. Tubercular arthritis.

8. A 12-year-old boy has complained of pain in his left groin at rest. His mother states that he has been limping and his school are becoming more concerned. There is no history of trauma.

9. A mother is concerned about her 3-month-old baby who has a clicking right hip. She has been finding it difficult to put nappies on due to limited movement at the hip.

10. A 3-year-old boy has been limping for 24 hours. He has been reluctant to put weight through his left leg. He has had recent viral upper respiratory tract infection, but is now well. A C-reactive protein (CRP) and white cell count are normal.

Paediatrics: *Multiple Choice Questions*

1. The Guthrie test in neonates screens for which of the following diseases? (select two options):
   - A. Phenylketonuria
   - B. Neonatal jaundice
   - C. Vitamin K deficiency
   - D. Congenital hyperthyroidism
   - E. Congenital hypothyroidism.

2. Which of the following is not a type of child abuse? (select one option only):
   - A. Physical
   - B. Failure to thrive
   - C. Neglect
   - D. Emotional
   - E. Sexual.

3. Which of the following is not considered a risk factor for child abuse? (select one option only):
   - A. Child with learning difficulties
   - B. Parent with substance misuse
   - C. Parental support network
   - D. Poor parental relationship
   - E. Poverty.

4. A 13-year-old boy is brought to A&E by his mother. He is drowsy and talking, but unable to give any history. His mother reports a '24 hour tummy bug' which caused diarrhoea and vomiting. He is tachycardic, hyperventilating and has a sweet smelling breath. Which of the following

will be your next step in managing this patient? (select one option only):

    A. Check the pupils
    B. Perform urine dipstick
    C. Secure IV access
    D. Perform ECG
    E. Perform CXR (chest x-ray).

5. A 4-year-old boy is brought in with paroxysmal abdominal colic which is becoming increasingly frequent. He has been vomiting and is crying in pain. You feel a sausage-shaped mass in the right upper quadrant on examination of his abdomen. Which of the following is the most likely diagnosis? (select one option only):

    A. Pyloric stenosis
    B. Urinary tract infection
    C. Gastroenteritis
    D. Intussusception
    E. Duodenal atresia.

Paediatrics: *Extended Matching Questions*

For each of the following scenarios, choose the most likely age at which the vaccination should be given (each option may be selected once, more than once or not at all):

    A. Soon after birth
    B. 2 months
    C. 3 months
    D. 4 months
    E. 12 months
    F. 13 months
    G. 10–14 years
    H. 12–13 years.

6. BCG vaccine to a newborn at high risk of tuberculosis (TB).

7. HPV vaccine against risk of cervical cancer.

8. First dose of MMR.

For each of the following, choose the most likely age at which a normal child should achieve the stated milestone (each option may be selected once, more than once or not at all):

    A. 6 weeks
    B. 3 months
    C. 6 months
    D. 9 months
    E. 12 months
    F. 15 months
    G. 18 months
    H. 2 years
    I. 3 years
    J. 4 years.

9. No head lag when pulled to sitting position.

10. Can get to standing position and walk.

11. Dry by day and night

Pharmacology/therapeutics: *Multiple Choice Questions*

1. A 70-year-old female who is on long-term prednisolone develops symptoms of cystitis. She is prescribed an antibiotic course during which she develops bilateral calf pain radiating to the heels. Which antibiotic may have caused her symptoms? (select one option only):

    A. Amoxicillin
    B. Co-amoxiclav
    C. Ciprofloxacin
    D. Nitrofurantoin
    E. Trimethoprim.

2. Which of the following is an enzyme inducer? (select one option only):

    A. Phenytoin
    B. Sodium valproate
    C. Omeprazole
    D. Fluoxetine
    E. Cimetidine.

Pharmacology/therapeutics: *Extended Matching Questions*

For each of the following, choose the drug most likely to have caused the given side effect (each option may be selected once, more than once or not at all):

    A. Rifampicin
    B. Augmentin
    C. Ethionamide
    D. Isoniazid
    E. Pyrazinamide
    F. Pyridoxine
    G. Erythromycin
    H. Ethambutol
    I. Prednisolone
    J. Streptomycin.

3. Orange-red discolouration of urine and bodily secretions.
4. Peripheral neuritis in high doses or in patients with pyridoxine deficiency.
5. Optic neuritis and red/green colour blindness.

For each of the following, choose the drug most likely to have been taken during pregnancy which caused the adverse effect (each option may be selected once, more than once or not at all):

    A. Augmentin
    B. Diethylstilbestrol
    C. Tetracycline
    D. Phenytoin
    E. Clexane
    F. Warfarin
    G. Fluoxetine
    H. Lithium
    I. Thalidomide
    J. Ramipril.

6. A neonate with frontal bossing and hypoplastic saddle nose.
7. A neonate with a neural tube defect, cleft lip and palate.
8. A neonate with Ebstein's anomaly.

Psychiatry/neurology: *Multiple Choice Questions*

1. The wife of a 35-year-old male who had a fall 1 week previously while intoxicated requests a home visit. She is concerned that her husband had initially been very drowsy and took time off work. He has now become aggressive and confused. Which is the single most likely cause for his symptoms? (select one option only):

   A. Alcohol intoxication
   B. Extradural haemorrhage
   C. Subdural haemorrhage
   D. Subarachnoid haemorrhage
   E. Dementia.

2. When can a patient diagnosed as having a TIA (transient ischaemic attack) resume driving? (select one option only):

   A. No need to discontinue driving
   B. 1 month
   C. 2 months
   D. 6 months
   E. 1 year.

3. A 28-year-old male known to be epileptic has a seizure while awake. How long must he refrain from driving? (select one option only):

   A. No need to discontinue driving
   B. 1 month
   C. 2 months
   D. 6 months
   E. 1 year.

4. Which of the following is a screening tool appropriate for the grading of depression of a 35-year-old male? (select one option only):

   A. AMTS
   B. CAGE
   C. Edinburgh PND
   D. MMSE
   E. PHQ-9.

Psychiatry/neurology: *Extended Matching Questions*

For each of the following scenarios, choose from the diagnoses below (each option may be selected once, more than once or not at all):

    A. Dementia
    B. Delirium
    C. Depression
    D. Mania
    E. Munchausen's syndrome
    F. Obsessive compulsive disorder
    G. Agoraphobia
    H. Schizophrenia.

5. A 19-year-old male is arrested and placed under psychiatric services following an arson attack. He states, 'the television was taking my thoughts away and putting bad ones in, it told me to burn the car'.

6. An 81-year-old female was stopped by the police for driving erratically. She was disorientated, unable to recall where she was going. She was admitted to hospital. There was no evidence of infection and the 'confusion screen' was normal. She had an MMSE (Mini Mental State Examination) score of 18/30.

7. A 35-year-old male is accompanied by his wife who is concerned that he has spent all their life savings on a yellow sports car. On questioning, he appears cheerful, talkative and has poor insight.

For each of the following scenarios, choose your most appropriate diagnosis (each option may be selected once, more than once or not at all):

    A. Analgesia-related headache
    B. Cluster headache
    C. Glaucoma
    D. Migraine
    E. Idiopathic intracranial hypertension
    F. Subarachnoid haemorrhage
    G. Tension headache
    H. Temporal arteritis.

8. A 40-year-old male has been experiencing repeated attacks of severe pain behind his right eye with each episode lasting 30 minutes.

9. A 24-year-old female has a sudden onset of an occipital headache, described as though someone has kicked her in the back of the head.

10. A 40-year-old overweight female has headaches first thing in the morning that are eased by standing.

Renal/urology: *Multiple Choice Questions*

1. A 55-year-old diabetic has an estimated glomerular filtration rate (eGFR) of approximately 35 mL/min for 1 year. At what stage is his chronic kidney disease (CKD)? (select one option):

   A. Stage 1
   B. Stage 2
   C. Stage 3
   D. Stage 4
   E. Stage 5.

2. Which of the following is not excreted by the kidneys? (select one option):

   A. Digoxin
   B. Lithium
   C. Lactulose
   D. Omeprazole
   E. Warfarin.

3. A 55-year-old male has lower urinary tract symptoms that include urinary frequency, urgency and reduced force of stream. Investigation excludes cancer. Which of the following drugs can be used to reduce symptoms? (select one option only):

   A. Atenolol
   B. Bendroflumethiazide
   C. Doxazosin
   D. Losartan
   E. Ramipril.

Renal/urology: *Extended Matching Questions*

For each of the following scenarios, choose your most likely cause of acute kidney injury (each option may be selected once, more than once or not at all):

    A. Acute tubular necrosis
    B. Hypovolaemia
    C. Myeloma
    D. Malignant hypertension
    E. Renal artery stenosis
    F. Renal tract obstruction
    G. Urinary tract infection.

4. A 69-year-old male is hypotensive post-operatively following a right total hip replacement. His blood pressure has remained low with a haemoglobin drop from 13.5 to 11.5 g/L.

5. A 55-year-old male suspected of having angina undergoes an angiogram. Following the procedure, his renal function has deteriorated.

6. A 96-year-old male with an enlarged prostate gland goes into acute urinary retention and is catheterized. He is noted to have acute kidney injury.

For each of the following scenarios, choose your most appropriate diagnosis (each option may be selected once, more than once or not at all):

    A. Acute tubular necrosis
    B. Diabetic renovascular disease
    C. Haemolytic uraemic syndrome
    D. Nephrotic syndrome
    E. Nephritic syndrome
    F. Nephrilithiasis
    G. Renal artery stenosis
    H. Thrombotic thrombocytopenic purpura
    I. Urinary tract infection.

7. A 22-year-old female has noticed that she is passing urine more frequently and it is causing her some discomfort.

8. A 5-year-old girl has an upper respiratory tract infection and develops facial swelling around the

eyes. She is noted to be more lethargic and irritable. Investigation reveals proteinuria with low levels of albumin.

9. A 6-year-old boy has bloody diarrhoea following a recent barbeque and his mother notices that he is passing urine less frequently. Urine MC&S (microscopy, culture and sensitivity) shows blood and protein.

Reproductive (male and female): *Multiple Choice Questions*

1. A 23-year-old pregnant female has been getting aching pain in her hands and arm especially at night. She reports pins and needles over the thumb, index and middle fingers. Which is the single most likely cause for her symptoms? (select one option only):
    A. Cervical spondylosis
    B. Cubital tunnel syndrome
    C. Carpal tunnel syndrome
    D. Erb's palsy
    E. Ulnar nerve compression at Guyon's canal.

2. A 16-year-old male reports a sudden onset of pain in the right groin and lower abdomen. He has been finding it uncomfortable to walk. Which is the single most important diagnosis to exclude? (select one option only):
    A. Appendicitis
    B. Irritable bowel syndrome
    C. Reducible hernia
    D. Testicular torsion
    E. Epididymo-orchitis.

3. Which of the following is a recognized benefit of hormone replacement therapy? (select one option only):
    A. Reduced risk of colonic carcinoma
    B. Reduces osteoporosis
    C. Reduced risk of ovarian carcinoma
    D. Reduces the risk of dementia
    E. Reduced risk of ischaemic heart disease.

4. Which of the following is not associated with azoospermia? (select one option):
   A. Cystic fibrosis
   B. Anabolic steroid abuse
   C. Chemoradiotherapy
   D. Varicocele
   E. 47XXY.

5. What is the gestational limit for termination of pregnancy in the UK? (select one option):
   A. No limit
   B. 16 weeks
   C. 20 weeks
   D. 24 weeks
   E. 30 week
   F. Depends on situation.

6. Which of the following are recognized complications following surgical termination of pregnancy? (select two options):
   A. Altered taste
   B. Uterine perforation
   C. Rhinorrhoea
   D. Failure of ovulation
   E. Retained products of conception.

7. Which of the following is not a recognized treatment for erectile dysfunction:
   A. Phosphodiesterase inhibitors
   B. Apomorphine
   C. Vacuum devices
   D. Penile implants
   E. Beta-blockers.

Reproductive (male and female): *Extended Matching Questions*

For each of the following scenarios, choose your most appropriate form of contraception (each option may be selected once, more than once or not at all):

   A. Condoms
   B. Diaphragm

      C.   Progesterone-only pill
      D.   Combined oral contraceptive pill
      E.   Implanon
      F.   Rhythm method
      G.   IUS (intrauterine system)
      H.   Female sterilization.

8. A 22-year-old female who suffers migraines with aura is looking for an oral contraceptive.

9. A 25-year-old female who is a poor pill taker and is not keen on condoms is looking for long-term contraception. She has a history of chlamydia. She is not in a regular relationship and not considering children.

10. A 48-year-old female who is married is having heavy periods that cause her significant pain.

Respiratory: *Multiple Choice Questions*

1. A 26-year-old female with brittle asthma attends an emergency GP surgery breathless and unable to complete her sentences. Examination findings show that she has a respiratory rate of 28 and a tachycardia of 120/min. What would be the next appropriate investigation to help assess the severity of her asthma within the practice? (select one option).

      A.   Chest x-ray
      B.   Electrocardiography (ECG)
      C.   Peak expiratory flow rate (PEFR)
      D.   Spirometry
      E.   Arterial blood gas sampling.

2. An asthmatic presents with tachypnoea, tachycardia and a peak expiratory flow rate that is <50% of her best predicted. Which one option in the management of acute severe asthma is inappropriate?

      A.   Sit the patient up
      B.   Provide oxygen
      C.   Give nebulized saline
      D.   Give IV hydrocortisone or oral prednisolone
      E.   Call 999 if failure of response to initial treatment.

3. A 56-year-old female is on the ward following a hysterectomy with a background PCA (patient-controlled analgesia) running. She is slow to recover and is noted to have shallow breathing with a respiratory rate of six breaths/minute. She has equal pinpoint pupils and a BM of 4.5. What is the next most appropriate action? (select one option):

    A. Intramuscular glucagon
    B. Intravenous glucose
    C. Subcutaneous insulin
    D. Continue PCA
    E. Intravenous naloxone

4. Which is the most common type of bronchial carcinoma in the UK? (select one option):

    A. Small cell carcinoma
    B. Squamous cell carcinoma
    C. Adenocarcinoma
    D. Mesothelioma
    E. Pulmonary blastoma.

5. In the management of obstructive sleep apnoea, which of the following is advised? (select one option):

    A. Sleeping with the windows open
    B. Avoidance of tobacco and alcohol
    C. Increasing fluid intake
    D. Reducing the head of the bed
    E. Increasing weight.

6. Exposure to which of the following is a recognized cause of extrinsic allergic alveolitis? (select one option):

    A. Pollen
    B. Cat hair
    C. Bird droppings
    D. Atmospheric dust
    E. UV radiation.

7. A 35-year-old asthmatic has a FEV_1/FVC ratio of 65%. What is the type of defect?

    A. Mixed
    B. Normal
    C. Obstructive
    D. Restrictive
    E. Variant.

Respiratory: *Extended Matching Questions*

For each of the following scenarios, choose your most appropriate diagnosis (each option may be selected once, more than once or not at all):

A. Acute left ventricular failure
B. Adult respiratory distress syndrome
C. Amniotic fluid embolism
D. Anaphylaxis
E. Asthma
F. Infective exacerbation of COPD
G. Pulmonary embolism
H. Pneumonia
I. Pulmonary fibrosis.

8. A 55-year-old female is 4 days post left mastectomy and notices that she is feeling breathless. She has had a temperature of 38.2° with some vague right-sided back pain.

9. A 45-year-old smoker presents with increasing shortness of breath, productive cough and fever.

10. A 68-year-old female presents in the early hours with acute onset breathlessness, fatigue and cough with pink froth.

Answers

Cardiovascular

1. *Answer: B – Increased HDL*

   High-density lipoprotein (HDL) is responsible for transport of cholesterol from the tissues to the liver. HDL is anti-atherogenic and its concentration is inversely related to the risk of coronary artery disease.

2. *Answer: E – After at least six weeks*

   According to the latest Department for Transport (DFT) – DVLA medical guidelines, a primary PCI disqualifies a group 2 licence holder (Large Goods Vehicle/Passenger Carrying Vehicle) for 6 weeks provided the exercise/functional tests can be met and there are no other disqualifying conditions.

3. *Answer: B – Immediately resume CPR at 30:2*

   If a cardiac rhythm shows pulseless electrical activity then you should immediately resume cardiopulmonary resuscitation 30:2 (30 chest compressions, 2 breaths) as this is a non-shockable rhythm. You would then need to reassess the rhythm and look for reversible causes. Adrenaline should be given every 3–5 minutes and other drugs such as atropine, amiodarone and magnesium should be considered.

4. *Answer: B - Kerley Z lines*

   Kerley A, B and C lines are seen on a chest x-ray representing fluid or tissue in the interlobular lymphatics. They are a consequence of left ventricular failure or mitral stenosis. They can also be seen in pulmonary fibrosis, parasitic infection or lymphangitis carcinomatosa. All the other options are common features in left ventricular failure.

5. *Answer: C – Pulmonary oedema*

   The causes of pulmonary oedema are cardiovascular (LVF post myocardial infarction (MI) or ischaemic heart disease); acute respiratory distress syndrome (ARDS), fluid overload or following a head injury. In the elderly it can be difficult to distinguish between COPD, pneumonia and pulmonary oedema. They may be co-existent and clinical skills are required to differentiate the diagnoses and treatment. Some hospitals can measure B-type natriuretic peptide (BNP) levels, which are grossly elevated (>1000) in pulmonary oedema but negative (<100) if the heart is not involved.

6. *Answer: A – 2.5 for 3 months*

For a distal DVT at least 6-week anticoagulation is recommended which should be increased to 3 months if a proximal DVT is suspected.

7. *Answer: D - 2.5 for 6 months*

For patients with idiopathic veno-thrombo-embolism or permanent risk factors at least 6 months treatment is recommended.

8. *Answer: I – none of the above*

Warfarin is teratogenic and should not be given in the first trimester of pregnancy. Oral anticoagulants cross the placenta and increase the risk of congenital malformations, placental/fetal and neonatal haemorrhage. Heparin does not cross the placenta. Lower molecular weight heparins such as enoxaparin are preferred due to ease of administration, reduced risk of osteoporosis and lower rates of heparin induced thrombocytopenia.

9. *Answer: A – Investigate for underlying cause.*

Higher readings in young patients require investigations for a secondary cause of hypertension including physical examination to assess for coarctation, blood tests assessing renal and thyroid function, renal ultrasound (to exclude renal artery stenosis), 24-hour urine collection for catecholamines (to exclude phaeochromocytoma) and cortisol levels (to exclude Cushing syndrome). Typically, patients are referred routinely for further investigations. Repeated high measurements are required to make a diagnosis. Ambulatory BP assessment can determine true hypertension versus white coat hypertension.

10. *Answer B – Urgent treatment and referral needed*

Whilst this is likely to be a response to her medication being stopped, this is a dangerously high BP and this patient should be referred urgently to a medical team for assessment and treatment.

11. *Answer F – Reassess annually*

Without further information regarding the patient's risk factors and history, you should respond with the safest and most appropriate option available. Reassessing blood pressure after 1 year is a reasonable response to a normal BP reading in a middle aged man.

12. *Answer: D - Myocardial infarction*

Cocaine use can cause myocardial infarction through a variety of mechanisms that include coronary artery vasospasm, an increased heart rate and blood pressure and the presence of a pro-thrombotic state.

13. *Answer: B – Decubitus angina*

Decubitus angina is a variant of angina pectoris that occurs while the patient is lying flat. It is theorized that this is due to an increase in myocardial oxygen demand caused by increased venous return whilst lying flat.

14. *Answer: F – Acute pericarditis*

Acute pericarditis is inflammation of the pericardium that typically presents with sharp central chest pain that is worse on inspiration or lying flat and relieved by sitting forward. ECG classically shows widespread saddle-shaped ST segment elevation. Treatment often involves identifying and treating a cause and the use of anti-inflammatory analgesia (e.g. ibuprofen).

DERMATOLOGY / ENT / EYE

1. *Answer: C – Basal cell carcinoma*

Basal cell carcinoma (rodent ulcer) is the most common malignant skin tumour usually affecting the middle-aged or elderly population. It has a predilection for sun-exposed areas such as the face, behind the ears and the upper trunk. The initial lesion is a small pearly-white nodule with visible telangiectatic blood vessels on the surface. The lesion may then bleed and ulcerate before healing. Management usually comprises excision, biopsy and radiotherapy.

2. Answer: C – Acute otitis media

Acute otitis media is common amongst infants and toddlers. It is typically viral and self-limiting. It tends to follow a viral upper respiratory tract infection and the Eustachian tube permits ascending infection. Bacterial superinfection follows leading to a more severe ear pain, fevers and the risk of eardrum perforation. Mastoiditis and meningitis are rare complications.

3. Answer: E – Eczema

Nasal polyps typically present in adulthood and are more common in males. Symptoms of presentation in progressive nasal obstruction, rhinorrhoea, post nasal drip, anosmia and sneezing. They are known to have an association with allergic rhinitis, aspirin sensitivity, chronic ethmoidal sinusitis and in children cystic fibrosis. The management of polyps involves testing for allergy, testing for cystic fibrosis in children and biopsying a unilateral polyp to exclude neoplasia.

4. Answer: D – Not to inform the DVLA and can drive

According to the latest DVLA medical guidelines notification of colour blindness is not necessary and driving can continue with no restriction for both group 1 and group 2 licences.

5. Answer: E – None of the above

These are all features of hypertensive retinopathy, which is classified into two groups. (1) Compensated hypertensive retinopathy describes AV nipping (arteriovenous crossings) and silver wiring (increased opacity and heightened light reflex). (2) Accelerated hypertensive retinopathy encompasses the cotton wool spots (retinal infarcts), flame haemorrhages, hard exudates and papilloedema.

6. Answer: C – Once every year

Diabetic retinopathy is a microvascular complication that increases the risk of blindness. National Institute of Health and Clinical Excellence (NICE) guidance suggests that routine review should take place yearly with earlier reviews if needed and appropriate timely referral to an ophthalmologist.

7. Answers: C and D – Eyelid hygiene and topical choramphenicol

Bacterial conjunctivitis is common and presents with an acute onset of grittiness and discharge. Examination may reveal crusty eyelid margins, mucopurulent discharge and conjunctival injection away from the limbus. Initial management involves eyelid hygiene and topical antibiotics.

8. *Answer: B – Atopic eczema*

Atopic eczema frequently appears in the first year of life, often resolving in early childhood. The eczema is generalized with the skin being dry and very itchy. Emollients are essential in the management of dry skin and topical steroids can be used to control severe inflammation. You should always consider and promptly treat secondary bacterial infection.

9. *Answer: E – Trigeminal zoster*

The trigeminal nerve consists of three main branches (ophthalmic, maxillary and mandibular). Herpes zoster can affect any of these divisions but the ophthalmic division is the most commonly affected. The skin eruption may be preceded by pain and usually consists of grouped vesicles on an erythematous base. The eruption normally resolves within 2 weeks, but patients may be troubled by post-herpetic neuralgia.

10. *Answer: G - Intertrigo*

'Intertrigo' is the term used to describe maceration that occurs when two skin surfaces are in apposition and associated moisture, friction or warmth is present. Most common sites include the groin, axillae, sub-mammary region. There is often added Candida infection. Treatment involves using a topical preparation of hydrocortisone and miconazole with attention being paid to hygiene.

11. *Answer: B - Pruritus gravidarum.*

This is also known as obstetric cholestasis or intrahepatic cholestasis of pregnancy. It occurs in 20% of pregnant women. The aetiology is unknown. It can be characterized by sudden onset of pruritis without any skin lesions. The palms and soles are commonly affected. 80% of cases occur during the third trimester. There is no effective treatment so expert input is advised early. Mild symptoms can be managed with soothing baths, emollients and oral anti-histamines.

12. *Answer: A – Polymorphic eruption of pregnancy*

Polymorphic eruption of pregnancy is a condition that usually occurs in first pregnancy. It often develops in the last trimester.

It is characterized as being an extremely pruritic condition that begins within abdominal striae, but often sparing the umbilicus. The lesions may spread to affect the trunk, arms and legs. It resolves shortly after delivery of the baby.

13. Answer: E – Varicella zoster

Varicella zoster (chickenpox) is spread by respiratory droplets and contact with vesicle fluid. It has an incubation period of 10-21 days and is infectious until all vesicles are crusted. It can present with fever, malaise and a maculopapular rash that becomes vesicular then crusts over. During pregnancy varicella can have serious implications for both mother and child. Maternal risk is increased because of increased susceptibility to varicella pneumonia, hepatitis and encephalitis. Fetal infection can happen in any trimester. If < 20 weeks gestation, there is a small risk of fetal varicella syndrome (congenital defects – skin scarring, limb hypoplasia, eye lesions and neurological abnormalities). Neonatal infection is seen if varicella is contracted in the last four weeks of pregnancy with severe infection being fatal.

14. Answer: A – Measles

Measles is caused by an RNA paramyxovirus and is spread by airborne or droplet transmission. It has an incubation period of 10-14 days. There is a prodromal stage characterized by the onset of fever, malaise, coryza, conjunctivitis and cough. After about 3 or 4 days there is the appearance of an erythematous maculopapular rash. White spots known as Koplik spots may be seen on the mucous membranes of the mouth. In the UK measles is a notifiable disease.

15. Answer: C – Rubella

Rubella (German Measles) is caused by infection with the Rubella virus (a rubivirus, of the family Togaviridae). This is spread by respiratory tract droplets. It has an incubation period of 14–21 days. In young children there are often no prodromal symptoms. A pink macular rash is seen in 50–80% of people that develops over two days and resolves by day four. There may also be associated cervical lymphadenopathy and arthralgia. The important complication of Rubella is the teratogenic effects of the virus during the first trimester of pregnancy.

16. *Answer: D – Meningococcal meningitis*

Meningococcal meningitis has an incubation period from 2 to 7 days and may have an insidious onset. Early features are often non-specific and include malaise, pyrexia and vomiting. There may be symptoms of headache, neck stiffness, photophobia and drowsiness. The development of a rash heralds meningococcal septicaemia. Therefore early recognition of the meningitis syndrome is important.

17. *Answer: A – Barotrauma*

Otic barotrauma is most often due to aircraft descent. It arises due to a difference between middle ear and ambient pressure. This may cause rupture of superficial vessels in the middle ear. It presents with acute pain, hearing loss and sensation of pressure in one or both ears. The aim is to equalise the pressure by yawning or sucking sweets.

18. *Answer: E – Menière's disease*

Menière's disease is a syndrome that usually affects only one ear and is characterised by a triad of vertigo, hearing loss and tinnitus. There is great variability in frequency and duration of episodes. First-line management is medical – avoidance of trigger factors and regular betahistine hydrochloride.

19. *Answer: G – Presbyacusis*

Presbyacusis is age-related sensorineural hearing loss that is progressive. It is common after the age of 55 and is a consequence of both a decline in the number of cochlea hair cells and degeneration of the cochlea nerve. There is a characteristic loss of high frequency sound perception making it difficult to understand speech.

20. *Answer: C - Monospot testing*

Glandular fever (infectious mononucleosis) is usually a self-limiting disease caused by the Epstein–Barr virus (EBV). It is commonly seen between the ages of 15 and 25 years. The incubation period is anywhere between four and eight weeks. There are a triad of symptoms that include fever, sore throat and lymphadenopathy. A positive Monospot (Paul Bunnell reaction) is seen in 90% of cases.

21. *Answer: E – Referral for IV antibiotics*

Quinsy is a complication of acute tonsillitis that can result in referred pain to the ear, severe dysphagia and trismus. There is a collection of pus on the outer capsule of the tonsil. The management often involves systemic antibiotics +/- surgical drainage.

22. *Answer: D – HIV testing*

HIV infection with seroconversion is classically seen after two to six weeks of exposure. This is the period where the virus is disseminating throughout the body. The clinical features of HIV seroconversion are many. Those commonly seen are sore throat, fever, lymphadenopathy, arthralgia and myalagia.

23. *Answer: C – Acute glaucoma*

Acute closed angle glaucoma occurs when there is an increase in intra-ocular pressure due to an impairment of aqueous outflow. This is due to a narrowing of the angle between the iris and trabecular meshwork at the entrance to the canal of Schlemm. The presentation is usually with an acutely painful red eye +/- loss of vision +/- nausea and vomiting. Examination reveals a semi-dilated, non-reacting pupil with a hazy cornea.

24. *Answer: H – Hypopyon*

Hypopyon is the presence of pus cells in the anterior chamber of the eye. It can often be seen following a bacterial infection or severe episode of iritis. There may be prior use of topical steroids or immunosuppression. Examination reveals a congested eye with evidence of prior iritis and a white/yellow fluid level of pus.

25. *Answer: F – Central retinal artery occlusion*

Central retinal artery occlusion presents with sudden painless loss of vision. It is uncommon and usually affects the elderly. The affected pupil is poorly reactive to light with the retina looking pale and oedematous. There is a characteristic "cherry red spot" over the fovea.

ENDOCRINOLOGY / METABOLIC

1. *Answer: D – ≥ 11.1*

   According to the World Health Organization (WHO) criteria, diabetes mellitus can be diagnosed if a patient has symptoms of hyperglycaemia (e.g. polyuria, polydipsia, unexplained weight loss, lethargy, genital thrush) AND a raised venous glucose detected once – fasting ≥ 7 mmol/L or random ≥11.1. Diagnosis can also be made using a raised venous glucose detected on two separate occasions (fasting level ≥ 7, or a random level ≥ 11.1). If there are any doubts, an oral glucose tolerance test (OGTT) should be organised to look for a 2-hour value >11.1.

2. *Answer: B – Start a biguanide*

   Metformin is the first line drug of choice to start in any overweight patient with Type 2 diabetes, provided there are no other contra-indications. The advantage of metformin is that it causes significantly less weight gain than some other hypoglycaemics.

3. *Answer: B – Oxytocin*

   The posterior pituitary gland secretes both oxytocin and vasopressin (ADH). Oxytocin plays an important role in female reproduction to facilitate both birth and breastfeeding.

4. *Answer: D - Exercise*

   Type 2 diabetes is becoming more prevalent largely to a change in lifestyle, better diagnosis and management. Reduced insulin secretion and insulin resistance is seen. It is associated with obesity and lack of exercise.

5. *Answer: H – Sheehan syndrome*

   Sheehan syndrome can cause post-partum hypopituitarism, due to post-partum haemorrhage which can significantly lower blood pressure and arrest the blood supply to the anterior pituitary, leading to infarction. The presentation can be variable and often includes failure of lactation, fatigue, loss of vigour and failure to resume normal menstruation. Treatment involves hormone replacement.

6. *Answer: I – Phaeochromocytoma*

   Phaeochromocytomas are tumours that arise from the adrenal medulla (chromaffin cells). There is usually a secretion of a combination of noradrenaline and adrenaline. Patients often present with high blood pressure and may have features related to catecholamine excess: headache, palpitations, tachycardia, sweating and anxiety. Stress is thought to be a trigger of an acute attack.

7. Answer: J – Cushing syndrome

Cushing syndrome results from chronic glucocorticoid excess with the commonest cause being steroid treatment. Endogenous causes are rare and include pituitary adenoma (Cushing disease) or a secreting adrenal adenoma (Cushing syndrome). Patients will often report weight gain, mood change, weakness and in women irregular menses, acne and hirsutism. Clinically you may find central obesity, moon face, buffalo hump, thin skin and purple abdominal striae. Management involves identifying and treating the cause.

8. Answer K – Levothyroxine

This presentation and blood investigations point towards a diagnosis of hypothyroidism. Symptoms are often subtle and the onset can be insidious with patients often reporting tiredness, lethargy, depression, intolerance of cold, weight gain, constipation and menorrhagia. The management involves replacement with levothyroxine.

9. Answer: I – Propylthiouracil

Thyrotoxicosis can occur during pregnancy with the commonest cause being Grave disease (autoimmune disease with production of TSH receptor stimulating antibodies). Early recognition and management improves maternal and fetal outcome. The treatment of choice for new cases during pregnancy is propylthiouracil as there is less transfer across the placenta and into breast milk when compared to carbimazole.

10. Answer: E – Metformin

The likely diagnosis here is polycystic ovary syndrome (PCOS). PCOS is associated with metabolic abnormalities that include insulin resistance and abnormal serum lipids. LH to FSH ratio is typically 3:1. Women should initially be encouraged to lose weight to lower this insulin resistance. Metformin can be utilised to increase insulin sensitivity.

GASTROENTEROGLOGY / NUTRITION

1. *Answer: B – Urgent referral for oesophago-gastro-duodenoscopy*

   Anyone over the age of 55 years with ALARM symptoms (Anaemia, Loss of weight, Anorexia, Recent onset of progressive symptoms, Malaena or swallowing difficulties) should be referred urgently for further investigation of the upper digestive tract.

2. *Answer: C – Irritable bowel syndrome*

   Irritable bowel syndrome (IBS) is a diagnosis of exclusion and used to describe abdominal symptoms for which no organic cause is found. Patients are often young and present with a multitude of symptoms that are chronic. Stress and menstruation are exacerbating factors. Management involves exclusion of other diagnoses and then symptom control. Referral may be appropriate.

3. *Answer: A – Ulcerative colitis*

   Ulcerative colitis is a relapsing and remitting inflammatory disorder confined to the large bowel. Patients experience cramping abdominal pain and diarrhoea that may be bloody. Medical management is the mainstay with surgery being reserved for emergencies (haemorrhage, perforation, toxic megacolon, colonic carcinoma) or where there are intractable symptoms.

4. *Answer: D – Primary biliary cirrhosis*

   Primary biliary cirrhosis is a progressive disease of the liver that is classically seen in middle-aged women. Half of patients may be asymptomatic whilst others have pruritus and fatigue. Jaundice and abdominal pain are features seen later as the disease progresses. Management involves symptom control and ultimately may need liver transplantation.

5. *Answer: D – Prostate-specific antigen*

   Prostate-specific antigen (PSA) is used in conjunction with symptoms for the diagnosis and monitoring of prostate carcinoma. PSA is sensitive but lacks specificity to be a 'stand-alone' test for prostate carcinoma as it can be elevated by other causes such as old age, benign prostatic enlargement, prostatitis, urine retention, following ejaculation and digital rectal examination.

6. *Answer: E – Calcitonin*

The underlying diagnosis here is likely to be medullary thyroid carcinoma, which arises from the parafollicular or C-cells of the thyroid gland. Calcitonin levels are often raised and diagnostic. High levels can cause nausea, vomiting, diarrhoea, flushing and altered sensation. There can be a familial association with 20% of medullary thyroid carcinomas occurring as part of the MEN-II syndrome.

7. *Answer: I – CA 125*

CA 125 is a tumour marker associated with ovarian cancer. It is elevated in 80% of women with advance disease but in early disease may be normal in 50% of patients.

8. *Answer: K – Urgent referral to surgical team*

The concern here is bowel obstruction and prompt referral to the surgical team is needed. Obstruction is classified according to location (small bowel or large bowel) and the causes whether mechanical or non-mechanical (paralytic ileus). Cardinal symptoms include vomiting, distension, absolute constipation and colicky abdominal pain. Management involves placing a nasogastric tube and maintaining hydration with intravenous fluids (the 'drip and suck' approach).

9. *Answer: A – Urine dipstick*

Here the most appropriate action would be to perform urinalysis to screen for a urinary tract infection and exclude pregnancy. You may still wish to send the urine sample off for microscopy, culture and sensitivity.

10. *Answer: I – Reassure*

The likely diagnosis here is either a bleeding haemorrhoid or an anal fissure. You can reassure the patient and advise a well balanced diet with plenty of fruit and fluids. Laxatives may have a role in keeping the stool soft so that it is easily passed.

INFECTIOUS DISEASE / HAEMATOLOGY / IMMUNOLOGY / GENETICS

1. *Answer: C – Erythromycin*

   According to the World Health Organization both erythromycin and azithromycin are suitable for the treatment of Chlamydia during pregnancy. However in the United Kingdom the use of azithromycin for the treatment of Chlamydia is not licensed.

2. *Answer: C – Iron deficiency anaemia*

   Iron deficiency classically produces a microcytic, hypochromic anaemia due to impaired erythropoiesis.

3. *Answers: A – High maternal age*

   Down syndrome is the commonest chromosomal disorder and its incidence increases with maternal age.

4. *Answer: B – 400 μg daily*

   Folic acid is important in the prevention of neural tube defects. It is vital to take supplements prior to conception. The usual dose is 400 μg daily, but this should be increased to 5 mg daily for women on anti-epileptic medication or to prevent a recurrence.

5. *Answers: A and C – Rubella and BCG*

   Rubella immunisation is given as part of the MMR vaccine that contains live-attenuated strains of measles, mumps and rubella. The BCG (bacillus Calmette–Guèrin) vaccine is also a live-attenuated strain of mycobacterium tuberculosis.

6. *Answer: B – Parvovirus*

   Parvovirus B19 (Fifth's disease) is often asymptomatic but can present with a typical 'slapped cheek' rash (erythema infectiosum), fever and arthralgia. There is significant risk to the fetus as the virus can suppress red cell production and is directly toxic to the heart. This results in heart failure and hydrops fetalis.

7. *Answer: B – Autosomal recessive*

   Cystic fibrosis is a common autosomal recessive disorder found in Caucasian populations. The cause is a mutation in the CF transmembrane conductance regulator (CFTR) gene on chromosome 7 that leads to defective chloride secretion and increased sodium absorption. These changes to the airway surface predispose the lung to chronic infections and bronchiectasis. Diagnosis is made via a sweat test looking for sweat sodium and chloride > 60 mmol/L.

8. *Answer: C – 300 µg intramuscular of 1:1000 adrenaline*

Anaphylactic shock is a medical emergency and time is of the essence. You should call for help and take an Airway, Breathing, Circulation and Disability, Exposure approach. Adrenaline should be administered if available with the dose for children aged 6–12 years being 300 µg intramuscularly of 1:1000 adrenaline. Adults should receive 500 µg IM of 1:1000 adrenaline.

9. *Answer: C – 1 in 2 risk of having an affected son*

The patient is a carrier of a recessive gene on one of her X chromosomes – marked as (h) in the grid below. Therefore, there is a 1:2 (50%) chance of any child inheriting this gene (and chromosome) provided her partner has only normal genes. Half of all sons would have the (h) gene.

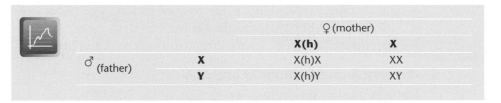

			♀ (mother)	
			X(h)	**X**
♂ (father)		**X**	X(h)X	XX
		Y	X(h)Y	XY

10. *Answer: B – Anticipation*

Genetic anticipation is the phenomenon where the signs and symptoms of a genetic condition appears earlier and is more severe in successive generations. Anticipation is more common in tri-nucleotide repeat disorders, e.g. Huntington's chorea and myotonic dystrophy.

11. *Answer: B, E and J – Chicken pox, Infectious mononucleosis and Schistosomiasis*

There are certain diseases that are notifiable to the consultant responsible for Communicable Disease Control under the public health Act 1984. Chicken pox, infectious mononucleosis and schistosomiasis are not included on this list.

12. *Answer: G – Bacterial vaginosis*

Bacterial vaginosis (BV) is not considered a sexually transmitted disease. It occurs due to an alteration in the normal vaginal bacterial flora. There is overgrowth of organisms such as Gardnerella vaginalis, Mobiluncus sp, Mycoplasma hominis and reduction in the normal lactobacillae. Diagnosis is based on the Amsel criteria: white adherent discharge, raised vaginal pH >4.5, release of fishy odour from the discharge with addition of potassium hydroxide and 'clue cells' on wet microscopy.

13. Answer: C – Candida

Candida is the commonest cause of vaginitis. This again is not a sexually transmitted disease but the risk factors include pregnancy, immunodeficiencies, diabetes, contraceptive pill and antibiotic use. Candida is classically described as a white curd-like discharge. There may also be surrounding vulval and vaginal irritation. Treatment is with the use of either a clotrimazole pessary, topical cream or oral fluconazole.

14. Answer: H – Trichomonas vaginalis

Trichomonas vaginalis is a sexually transmitted infection that produces a vaginitis and a profuse vaginal discharge. The discharge can be yellow or green and is often accompanied by an offensive smell. Clinically the vulva may appear red and swollen, with a 'strawberry cervix'. Diagnosis is by identifying motile flagellate on a wet film microscopy. Treatment is with Metronidazole.

15. Answer: C – Pernicious anaemia

Pernicious anaemia is an autoimmune disease that is causes an atrophic gastritis leading to a lack of gastric intrinsic factor. Intrinsic factor is involved in the absorption of vitamin B_{12} in the terminal ileum. B_{12} is important in the synthesis of DNA and consequentially red blood cell production is impaired.

16. Answer: G Aplastic anaemia

Aplastic anaemia is a rare condition that presents with anaemia, bleeding and recurrent bacterial infections. The exact cause is unknown but it is thought to be largely acquired and may result from defects of haemopoietic stem cells. An analysis of the peripheral blood film and bone marrow is used for diagnosis. Prognosis usually depends upon the cause and is poor.

17. Answer: D – Iron deficiency anaemia

Iron deficiency anaemia is common. The causes in a postmenopausal woman may include poor dietary intake of iron, malabsorption, malignancy and gastrointestinal blood loss. Patients may present with koilonychias, atrophic glossitis and angular stomatitis. A rare complication is Plummer–Vinson syndrome where there is development of post-cricoid webs that cause dysphagia. The best test for iron deficiency anaemia is serum ferritin that is low. The total iron binding capacity is increased. Management involves identifying an underlying cause and replacing iron either with supplements or through dietary changes.

18. Answer: B – 45 XO

Turner's syndrome (45 XO) is a condition seen in females where there is gonadal hypoplasia and a range of somatic features that include webbed neck, widely spaced nipples, cubitus valgus, low set ears and hypertension. There are no secondary sexual characteristics. Affected girls are usually of a short stature, infertile and have primary amenorrhoea. Early diagnosis is important as it enables hormone replacement therapy.

19. Answer: G – 47 XXY

Klinefelter's syndrome (47 XXY) is a cause of male hypogonadism. Patients may be tall, have prominent gynaecomastia and exhibit behavioural disorders. They often show normal masculinization and may only have infertility.

20. Answer: H – Trisomy 18

Edward's syndrome (Trisomy 18) is a rare cause of mental retardation. It is the second most common trisomy that survives to term after Down syndrome. There is a characteristic facies that includes microcephaly, low set ears and a crowded face with micrognathia. There are also limb problems with flexed fingers, overlapping of index and little finger and rocker-bottom feet. Patau syndrome (trisomy 13) typically results from an error in meiosis. This also features rocker-bottom feet and low set ears but the condition is much more rare and survival beyond a few weeks is rare. Polydactyly is a common feature.

MUSCULOSKELETAL

1. Answer: C – Colles' fracture

A Colles' fracture is an injury of the distal end of the radius within 2.5 cm of the wrist. There is dorsal (posterior) angulation of the distal fractured fragment and you may see the characteristic "dinner fork" deformity. This classically results from a fall onto an outstretched hand.

A Smith's fracture is often referred to as a 'reverse Colles' fracture'. There is distal radial fracture that is impacted with volar (anterior) angulation of the distal fracture fragment. This usually results from a fall onto a flexed wrist.

A Barton's fracture is an intra-articular fracture of the distal radius only involving the volar (anterior) portion. The fracture is very unstable and most patients will require open reduction with internal fixation.

A Bennett's fracture-dislocation is an injury through the base of the first metacarpal (thumb) with radial subluxation. The injury results from a fall onto the thumb or a fall onto a closed fist around the thumb. It may need surgical fixation as it is an unstable injury and difficult to manage in a plaster of Paris (POP) cast.

A Jones' fracture is a transverse injury of the base of the fifth metatarsal. It is prone to poor healing and should be managed in a below-knee POP with orthopaedic follow up.

2. Answer: I – Myeloma

Myeloma is a malignant neoplasm of B-lymphocytes derived from plasma cells. The normal function of B-lymphocytes is to produce different immunoglobulins (polyclonal) but in myeloma a single cell has replicated in an abnormal manner (clonal) all producing identical immunoglobulin. This forms the basis of diagnosis with a monoclonal band or paraprotein. Presentation is with unexplained backache, pathological fracture, recurrent infections, lethargy and weight loss.

3. Answer: G – Cauda equina syndrome

Cauda equina syndrome occurs due to compression of the cauda equina nerve roots, which could be due to traumatic injury, disc herniation, abscess, epidural haematoma or neoplasm. Patients present with lower back pain radiating down one or both legs. They often notice lower extremity motor and/or sensory abnormality along with bladder and/or bowel dysfunction. The term 'saddle anaesthesia' is often used to describes reduced sensation in the perianal region. It is a neurological emergency.

4. Answer: H – Polymyalgia rheumatica

Polymyalgia rheumatica predominantly occurs in middle-aged to elderly women. Typical presentation is with stiffness and pain in the pectoral and pelvic girdles. Systemic features such as malaise, anorexia, low-grade fever, weight loss, depression and night sweats may also be present. There is elevation of acute inflammatory markers (CRP and ESR) and patient may have a normochromic normocytic anaemia. Treatment is with low dose steroids that should be titrated according to response.

5. Answer: C – Osteoarthritis

Osteoarthritis is the result of 'wear and tear' of the articular surface. Presentation is often with insidious onset of pain that progressively worsens over months. The pain is typically worse with exertion and relieved with rest. Early morning stiffness is classic after a long duration of rest. In severe cases there may be joint swelling and/or deformity. Early osteoarthritis can be managed symptomatically however advanced disease may require radical surgery or arthroplasty.

6. Answer: E – Septic arthritis

Septic arthritis is vital to diagnose and manage promptly to avoid joint destruction. Infection reaches a joint via the blood stream with the commonest pathogens being *Staphlyococcus aureus*, *Haemophilus*, *Gonococcus*, *Streptococcus*, TB and Salmonella. Clinical presentation is with a red, painful and swollen joint. Any movement at the joint causes significant pain and therefore it is held in a position of comfort. There may have been a prodrome of general malaise and increase temperature. Management involves urgent intravenous antibiotics and arthroscopic joint washout if necessary.

7. Answer: H – Pseudogout

Pseudogout is usually a condition of the elderly due to deposition of brick-shaped or rhomboid calcium pyrophosphate dihydrate (CPPD) crystals in a large joint. This deposition results in an acute synovitis with joint pain and swelling. X-rays may show the deposited CPPD and aspiration of the synovial fluid shows positively birefringent crystals. Management involves rest and anti-inflammatory drugs. There may be use of intra-articular corticosteroid injection. Note that gout has needle-shaped negatively birefringent crystals.

8. *Answer: E – Slipped upper femoral epiphysis (SUFE)*

Slipped upper femoral epiphysis (SUFE) is a condition that primarily affects boys between the ages of 10 and 15 years. There is usually posterior–inferior displacement of the upper femoral epiphysis against the femur. The exact cause is unknown but there is some association with obesity, delayed secondary sexual development and tall boys. Presentation is often with rest pain in the upper thigh or knee with occasional pain in the groin. Pain on movement and limp may also be a feature.

9. *Answer: B – Congenital dislocation of the hip (CDH)*

Congenital dislocation of the hip (CDH) is a spectrum of anomalies that results in unstable hips or subluxation. Screening is performed on the neonatal and the six week surveillance checks using the Ortolani and Barlow test.

10. *Answer: G – Transient synovitis*

Transient synovitis of the hip (irritable hip) is a diagnosis made only after exclusion of serious causes of hip pain e.g. septic arthritis, Perthes' disease, SUFE. It is the commonest cause of hip pain in children.

PAEDIATRICS

1. *Answers: A and E – Phenylketonuria and Congenital hypothyroidism*

As part of the newborn blood spot screening programme, a heel-prick blood test (Guthrie test) is undertaken for phenylketonuria and congenital hypothyroidism. It can also test for other diseases, such as sickle-cell or cystic fibrosis.

2. *Answer: B – Failure to thrive*

'Failure to thrive' is defined as a significant interruption in the expected rate of growth during childhood. This is a common problem in paediatric medicine and may reflect an underlying pathological process.

3. *Answer: C – Parental support network*

   You must be aware of the types of and risk factors for child abuse. Safeguarding children is fundamental. You should know the local policy in your Trust.

4. *Answer: C – Secure IV access*

   In diabetic ketoacidosis, recognition and diagnosis of the condition is paramount. Securing IV access and reversing the metabolic abnormalities with insulin and IV fluid is essential and is your priority.

5. *Answer: D – Intussusception*

   Failure to recognize and appropriately manage intussusception is fatal. It occurs when one portion of bowel 'telescopes' into the lumen of the adjoining bowel. Clinical presentation is variable and may include paroxysms of colicky abdominal pain, vomiting and passage of blood from the anus that is often described as 'redcurrant jelly'. The treatment of choice is reduction using barium enema. Surgery is indicated for young children or those aged over 2 years and if there are signs of either peritonism or gross dehydration.

6. *Answer: A – Soon after birth*

   BCG vaccination should be given soon after birth for all infants at high risk of TB (infants in areas of high TB prevalence or if their parents/grandparents born in a country of high TB incidence).

7. *Answer: H – 12-13 years*

   In the UK the HPV vaccine is targeted at girls from the ages of 12 and 13 years.

8. *Answer: F – 13 months*

   The first dose of the MMR vaccine is given at 13 months. The second dose is given three months after the first dose.

9. *Answer: C – 6 months*

   At 6 months, the head is controlled on the shoulders and there is no head lag when pulled to a sitting position.

10. *Answer: F – 15 months*

    At 15 months, the child is able to get to a standing position alone and can walk steadily with a broad based gait. They may, however, fall over.

11. *Answer: J – 4 years*

By four years of age a child is able to attend their entire toilet needs.

PHARMACOLOGY / THERAPEUTICS

1. *Answer: C – Ciprofloxacin*

Ciprofloxacin is linked with tendinopathy (tendinitis/tendon rupture). The exact mechanism is poorly understood. It is thought to both cause an increase in protease activity from fibroblasts, and exert an inhibitory effect on fibroblast metabolism

2. *Answer: A – Phenytoin*

Phenytoin is a hepatic enzyme inducer that may decrease the bioavailability of drugs that are metabolised by hepatic enzymes. Similarly it may increase the bioavailability of other drugs that require metabolism by hepatic enzymes for their activation.

3. *Answer: A – Rifampicin*

Rifampicin is a drug commonly used in the treatment of tuberculosis and in the prophylaxis of meningococcal meningitis. It is known to change the colour of bodily secretions to orange-red.

4. *Answer: D – Isoniazid*

Isoniazid is primarily used in the treatment of tuberculosis. In high doses or in patients with pyridoxine deficiency it can lead to peripheral neuritis.

5. *Answer: H – Ethambutol*

Ethambutol is used in drug-resistant tuberculosis. It can have profound visual side effects that include red/green colour blindness and optic neuritis.

6. *Answer: F – Warfarin*

Warfarin is teratogenic as it crosses the placenta. Its use can result in frontal bossing, hypoplasia, saddling of the nose, cardiac defects, short stature, blindness and mental retardation.

7. Answer: D – Phenytoin

Phenytoin has been suggested to cause a folate deficiency, which in turn increases the risks of neural tube defects during pregnancy. Pregnant women on anti-epileptic medication are advised to take a higher dose of daily folic acid supplements (5 mg once daily)

8. Answer: H – Lithium

Lithium during pregnancy increases the incidence of Ebstein anomaly. There is also an association with an increased risk of miscarriage. Ebstein anomaly is a congenital structural defect of the heart in which there is downward (apical) displacement of the tricuspid valve causing 'atrialization' of the right ventricle. There is often an atrial septal defect.

PSYCHIATRY / NEUROLOGY

1. Answer: C – Subdural haemorrhage

A subdural haemorrhage commonly results from a traumatic event. There is bleeding from the bridging veins between the cortex and the venous sinuses resulting in accumulation of blood. The presentation may vary from a fluctuating level of consciousness with insidious slowing (intellectual, physical) to a complete personality change.

2. Answer: B – 1 month

For any cerebrovascular disease (stroke, intracerebral haemorrhage, TIA, amaurosis fugax, intracranial venous thrombosis) driving may resume after 1 month provided there is satisfactory clinical recovery. There is no need to notify the DVLA unless a residual neurological deficit persists.

3. Answer: E – 1 year

A person who has suffered an epileptic attack whilst awake must refrain from driving for at least one year before a driving licence is issued.

4. Answer: E – PHQ-9

PHQ-9 is a validated depression assessment tool looking at each of the DSM-IV criteria for depression. It allows grading of depression severity based upon score.

5. Answer: H – Schizophrenia

Schizophrenia is a syndrome affecting all areas of a person's function, best described using Schneider's first rank symptoms. These include auditory hallucinations (third person auditory hallucinations in the form of a running commentary), thought withdrawal and/or thought insertion, thought broadcasting, delusional perceptions and somatic passivity.

6. Answer: A – Dementia

Dementia is a progressive and irreversible deterioration in intellectual function, behaviour and personality. Consciousness is not affected. There are many different subtypes (Alzheimer's disease, Lewy body, frontotemporal, vascular, Parkinson's and mixed) and efforts should be made to categorise using CT/MRI (computed tomography/magnetic resonance imaging) and SPECT (single photon emission computed tomography) imaging. Reversible causes such as hypothyroidism, B_{12} deficiency and syphilis should be sought and treated. Treatment involves managing symptoms and behaviours while addressing risk. Acetylcholinesterase inhibitors such as donepezil, galantamine and rivastigmine can be used in moderate Alzheimer's dementia (MMSE 10–20 points).

7. Answer: D – Mania

Mania is a disorder of mood resulting in feelings of elation and euphoria. Patients commonly have vast amounts of energy, are easily irritable, have flight of ideas, poor concentration, grandiose delusions and little or no insight.

8. Answer: B – Cluster headache

Cluster headaches present with very severe and localised pain around one of the orbits. It is more common in men and onset is usually in the 40s. The attacks occur in clusters of approximately 6–8 weeks. Management can prove to be extremely difficult and may necessitate referral to a neurologist.

9. Answer: F – Subarachnoid haemorrhage

Spontaneous rupture of a saccular aneurysm commonly causes a subarachnoid haemorrhage. Presentation is often with a sudden onset headache, typically in the occipital region. There may also be vomiting, collapse, seizure, drowsiness and more devastating, coma. The majority are due to a 'berry' aneurysm. Prognosis is variable and requires intensive management in a neurosurgical centre. IV fluids are given to maintain plasma volume and Nimodipine (60 mg 4 hourly) is given to prevent a secondary vasospasm of cranial arteries which can lead to delayed cerebral ischaemia.

10. Answer: E – Idiopathic (benign) intracranial hypertension

Idiopathic intracranial hypertension commonly occurs in women who are obese. The exact aetiology is unclear. The oral contraceptive pill is a recognised risk factor. Women often present with headache, noticeable either first thing in the morning or late at night. Leaning forward often exacerbates the headache. There may be transient visual disturbances and diplopia. Non-specific symptoms may include dizziness, nausea, vomiting, photopsia (flashes of light) and tinnitus. Treatment can involve serial therapeutic lumbar punctures to remove cerebrospinal fluid (CSF). Acetazolamide and thiazide diuretics may be used under supervision by a neurologist.

RENAL / UROLOGY

1. Answer: C – Stage 3

Chronic kidney disease is staged to allow for improved communication and defining thresholds for intervention. An eGFR of 35 mL/min corresponds to stage 3.

2. Answer: C – Lactulose

Lactulose is excreted through faeces. Drugs have three main routes of excretion from the body which include the urine, faeces and saliva. Renal excretion is by far the commonest.

3. Answer: C – Doxazosin

Doxazosin is an alpha-blocker that can be used to reduce smooth-muscle tension in the prostate, urethra and bladder neck thereby aiding passage of urine. This can be seen as a bridge to surgical intervention to resect the enlarged prostate gland.

4. Answer: B – Hypovolaemia

Hypovolaemia leads to renal hypoperfusion and is a pre-renal cause of acute kidney injury.

5. *Answer: A – Acute tubular necrosis*

Radiological contrast media are nephrotoxic and can cause acute tubular necrosis where there is direct damage to the renal tubular cells. This often recovers with conservative measures.

6. *Answer: F – Renal tract obstruction*

Obstructive uropathy due to the enlarged prostate gland leads to an inability to pass urine. The resultant increase in pressure within the collecting system and ureters increases the intratubal pressure within the kidney leading to acute kidney injury.

7. *Answer: I – Urinary tract infection*

A urinary tract infection is the presence of a pure growth of $>10^5$ organism per mL of urine. It can either be classified as uncomplicated (normal renal tract and function) or complicated (abnormal renal tract, immuno-compromised). The commonest organism implicated in the community is E.coli.

8. *Answer: D – Nephrotic syndrome*

Nephrotic syndrome is a triad of proteinuria (>3g/24hrs), hypoalbuminaemia (<30g/L) and oedema. The commonest cause is glomerulonephritis although the syndrome can be seen with diabetes, amyloidosis, systemic lupus erythematosus (SLE) and drugs reactions/allergies.

9. *Answer: C – Haemolytic uraemic syndrome*

Haemolytic uraemic syndrome consists of acute renal failure, microangiopathic haemolytic anaemia (MAHA) and thrombocytopenia. The majority of cases are due to E.coli 0157 (uncooked meat) that commonly affects young children who present with abdominal pain, bloody diarrhoea and oliguria.

REPRODUCTIVE (MALE & FEMALE)

1. *Answer: C – Carpal tunnel syndrome*

The median nerve is compressed under the flexor retinaculum. The muscle supply is recalled by 'LOAF': lateral two lumbricals, opponens pollicis, abductor pollicis brevis, flexor pollicis brevis. The median nerve supplies the palmar surface of the hand, however, the sensation can be intact because a palmar branch of the median nerve can pass superficial to the flexor retinaculum.

Women are predisposed and pregnancy and rheumatoid arthritis are the most common causes in young patients.

2. Answer: D – Testicular torsion

Testicular torsion is a surgical emergency. It is most common in adolescents, but can occur in all age groups. The scrotum is typically swollen and tender, with associated lower abdominal pain. Beware of testicular torsion in undescended testes.

3. Answer: B – Reduces osteoporosis

The benefits of hormone replacement therapy may include symptomatic relief of flushing, headaches and insomnia. There is also reversal of genital tract atrophy and reduced risk of osteoporosis. The evidence for reducing ischaemic heart disease is controversial and recent studies have suggested no benefit, and potentially harm occurs.

4. Answer: D – Varicocele

'Azoospermia' is the term used to describe the absence of sperm cells within the ejaculate. The causes can be defined as pretestiular (anabolic steroid abuse, Kalmann's, pituitary adenoma, hypogonadotrophic hypogonadism), non-obstructive (cryptorchidism, orchitis, 47 XXY, chemoradiotherapy) and obstructive (congenital absence of the vas deferens, vasectomy, sexually transmitted infections (STI))

5. Answer: D – 24 weeks

The gestational age for termination of pregnancy is situation dependant. Where the mother's life is threatened or there is risk of grave permanent physical or mental injury to the mother or risk of serious handicap to the child there is no gestational limit to termination of pregnancy.

6. Answer: B, E – uterine perforation and retained products of conception

Termination of pregnancy carries its own inherent complications that vary depending on the mode used. The main complications seen include bleeding, genital tract infections, uterine perforation/rupture, cervical trauma, failure of procedure, retained products of conception and long term psychological impact.

7. Answer: E – Beta blockers

Erectile dysfunction can occur at any age but is more common in middle age. The causes can be divided into organic (multiple sclerosis (MS), spinal cord damage, endocrine (e.g. diabetes), hypertension) and psychological (depression, relationship problems). Management can either include a pharmacological approach using phosphodiesterase 5 inhibitors (sildenafil, tadalafil), apomorphine dopamine agonist, or the use of devices to aid and maintain erection (vacuum devices and penile implants). Beta blockers are a common cause of erectile dysfunction.

8. Answer: C – Progesterone only pill

For a short-acting reversible contraceptive, consideration needs to be given to the contraceptive pill. According to the UK Medical Eligibility Criteria (UKMEC) migraine with aura is a UKMEC category 4 (represents an unacceptable health risk) for the combined oral contraceptive pill. The progesterone only pill would be a suitable choice as this is a UKMEC category 2 (advantages of using method outweighs the theoretical risk).

9. Answer: E – Implanon

Both Implanon and the intrauterine system offer long-term reversible contraception. The implanon is more suitable in this case, given that she has risk factors for pelvic infection. She should be advised to use condoms concurrently.

10. Answer: G – Intrauterine system

The intrauterine system (IUS) (e.g. Mirena coil) is ideal in this situation as it has been shown to reduce bleeding and the pain associated with menstruation. You must counsel patients regarding the possibility of initial increase in bleeding. The IUS will also provide her with contraception that she could potentially keep until she reaches the menopause.

RESPIRATORY

1. Answer: C – Peak expiratory flow rate

This is a medical emergency and this patient should be treated with salbutamol nebulisers and oxygen urgently. Whilst peak expiratory flow rate (PEFR) will help stratify the severity of the asthma attack, patients who cannot complete sentences, typically cannot manage an adequate 'blow' on the PEFR meter. Of the choices presented, PEFR is the most appropriate next step within the practice.

2. Answer: C – Give nebulised saline

The history above classifies asthma as acute severe. According to British Thoracic Society (BTS) guidelines for the management of asthma, initial management can take place in the primary care setting with oxygen and nebulized beta-2 bronchodilatation (salbutamol 5 mg). Steroids should also be given. If symptoms persist with any features of acute severe asthma after initial treatment the patient should be referred to A&E.

3. Answer: E - Intravenous naloxone

Opioid-induced respiratory depression needs reversal with naloxone which is a specific antidote. Naloxone has an impressively rapid onset of action but has a short half-life and will need to be repeated several times or set up via a continuous infusion. Caution should be used when administering naloxone in patients with severe or chronic pain, because it will reverse the analgesia effect of the opioid, potentially leaving the patient in agony. In a controlled situation, small aliquots can be given. However in the context of a respiratory emergency it is usual to give a full bolus.

4. Answer: B - Squamous cell carcinoma

Carcinoma of the bronchus is common, with cigarette smoking being the principle risk factor. The commonest type is squamous cell carcinoma accounting for approximately 40% of all cases; it has better prognosis than adenocarcinoma. It characteristically affects the large central bronchi and can rapidly grow to a large size. Physical compression of the bronchi can lead to lobar collapse, recurrent pneumonia, bronchiectasis and lung abscesses. Spread is via lymphatic and blood routes but does so late. Small cell carcinoma ('oat cell') accounts for 20-30% while adenocarcinoma accounts for 20% and large cell carcinoma for 10%. Small cell carcinoma is aggressive and poorly differentiated; it metastasises early. Adenocarcinoma is more common in non-smokers and following asbestos exposure.

5. *Answer: B - Avoidance of tobacco and alcohol*

Obstructive sleep apnoea is a disorder of breathing during sleep because of intermittent closure of the airways resulting in apnoeic episodes. It typically occurs in the obese with short necks. Spouses will report heavy snoring broken by breath-holding and apnoeic episodes. This rouses the patient leading to poor quality sleep. Classically there is daytime somnolence: the patient falls asleep easily when sitting in a chair or reading. Patients may fall asleep while driving. Management depends on the severity of the condition but simple management advice may include weight reduction, cessation of smoking, abstinence from alcohol, raising the head of the bed and sleeping for adequate periods of time. Referral to a sleep clinic can lead to definitive diagnosis. Nocturnal CPAP (continuous positive airway pressure) machines can revolutionise patients' lives.

6. *Answer: C - Bird droppings*

Extrinsic allergic alveolitis is a hypersensitivity reaction to an inhaled organic dust. This allergen commonly includes avian proteins found in bird dropping (bird/pigeon fancier's lung) and fungal spores such as aspergillus (farmer's/mushroom worker's and maltworker's lung). Classically the patient has dyspnoea, wheeze and cough with malaise, fever and myalgia within hours of exposure. Chronic exposure leads to pulmonary fibrosis. Allergy testing and eosophillia help diagnosis. Allergen avoidance is key to management.

7. *Answer: C - Obstructive*

The FEV_1/FVC gives an estimate of the airway calibre. If the ratio is decreased i.e. <75% then there is airway obstruction as seen in asthma or COPD.

8. *Answer: G – Pulmonary embolus.*

Pulmonary embolism requires a high degree of suspicion to make the diagnosis and should always be considered as a cause of post-operative breathlessness. Typically, a deep venous thrombus forms within the pelvis which can then shower through the venous circulation and the right side of the heart before settling within the pulmonary circulation. Risk factors include recent surgery, recent stroke, malignancy, immobility, pregnancy and contraceptive/HRT use. Saddle-shaped PEs can be catastrophic, lodging in the pulmonary artery causing acute cardiorespiratory collapse. Note that the temperature can be a red-herring, though a post-operative pneumonia should also be considered.

9. Answer: F – Infective exacerbation of COPD

Infective exacerbation of COPD is associated with dyspnoea and sputum production. Management involves the increased use of bronchodilators (inhalers, nebulizers), antibiotics and steroids. It is important to determine whether a patient can be managed in the community or requires hospital treatment. Factors favouring hospital treatment include inability to cope at home, severe breathlessness, confusion, impaired consciousness, long-term oxygen therapy (LTOT) use and significant co-morbidities.

10. Answer: A – Acute left ventricular failure

Acute left ventricular failure is a medical emergency that requires prompt diagnosis and treatment. The failure of the left ventricle to effectively eject blood in systole increases the end-diastolic volume and pressure in the left ventricle. This rapidly causes high left atrial pressure with fluid subsequently collecting in the alveoli. This impairs gas exchange leading to worsening dyspnoea. Immediate management involves prompt assessment and treating on clinical findings. This involves sitting the patient up, administering oxygen, GTN if blood pressure allows and then intravenous furosemide.

9 Professional dilemmas: questions and answers

Sukhjinder Nijjer and Rajesh Kumar

Question 1

You are an FY2 doctor on a cardiology rotation in hospital. You are with a family who are complaining about the sudden death of their 23-year-old son who was recently diagnosed with a cardiomyopathy. Your bleep goes off. It is a nurse requesting your immediate assistance for a patient who is complaining of crushing central chest pain. What do you do?

Rank the following in order (1, most appropriate; 4, least appropriate)

A. Tell the nurse you are busy and that you will not attend.
B. Ask a colleague within your team to see the patient with chest pain, while you wrap up with the family and will then join your colleague.
C. Apologise to the family, inform them that you have an emergency to deal with and request a short break while you attend to the patient.
D. Leave the family without telling them or informing anyone else.

Enter your answer:

1st	
2nd	
3rd	
4th	

Suggested answer 1

The key issues to consider in this scenario are patient safety, dealing with complaints and asking for help from colleagues.

Option A is least appropriate, as this is entirely unacceptable management for a patient with chest pain. It is also unprofessional because you are dismissing the nurse's concerns about the patient and putting patient safety at risk.

Option B is most appropriate because you are dealing with both the chest pain patient and minimizing the disruption caused to the family who are complaining to you.

Option C is another appropriate option. However, you do not know how long it will take for you to manage the chest pain patient, so the family may be waiting a while.

Option D addresses the patient safety issue, but results in the family being left unaware of your whereabouts – which is likely to fuel further complaint.

Given this information the most appropriate order would be:

1st	B
2nd	C
3rd	D
4th	A

Question 2

You are an SHO on an elderly care rotation. During your morning ward round, an elderly patient with mild dementia tells you that her treasured gold watch has gone missing from her bedside locker. She accuses the nursing staff. How would you respond?

Rank the following in order (1, most appropriate; 5, least appropriate)

A. Tell the patient that she is senile and the nurses would have no interest in stealing her watch.
B. Ask the patient for a description of her watch and when she last saw it, and inform her that you will deal with it.
C. Go to the nurses' station and demand that the nurses return the patient's watch.
D. Contact the police.
E. Discuss the issue in this afternoon's MDT meeting.

Enter your answer:

1st	
2nd	
3rd	
4th	
5th	

Suggested answer 2

This scenario deals with:

- Addressing patient concerns
- Avoiding discrimination
- Assumptions of staff involvement
- Judged severity of crime.

Option A is very inappropriate because it is unprofessional, very rude and patronizing to the patient.

Option B is very appropriate as you can establish the exact details of what has gone missing so that it will help in recovering the items.

Option C jumps to the conclusion that a member of nursing staff has stolen the watch. It is unlikely that any thief would return the missing items for fear of being identified. It is also equally possible that an outsider such as a ward visitor is responsible. In any case this is counterproductive to the team dynamic and may cause conflict.

Option D seems very unreasonable, as we have not established if the items have been misplaced or stolen, or if they were even present in the first place. If controlled drugs had gone missing then there would be a stronger case to get the police involved.

Option E is appropriate as it may allow some facts to be established and addresses the patient's concern. It would also create a heightened level of awareness and allows staff to be more vigilant.

Given this information the most appropriate order would be:

1st	B
2nd	E
3rd	C
4th	D
5th	A

Question 3

You are an FY2 doctor on the medical assessment unit. On the busy post-take ward round, the registrar prescribes trimethoprim for a urinary tract infection on a fresh drug chart. He does not enquire about allergies. You are later bleeped by the pharmacist who informs you that the patient is allergic to trimethoprim. What action do you take?

Choose the three most appropriate actions:

    A. Apologise and amend the prescription with an appropriate alternative.
    B. Do nothing.
    C. Blame one of the nurses for saying the patient had no allergies.
    D. Call the registrar to the ward immediately and ask them to explain their actions to the pharmacist.
    E. Report the incident directly to the clinical director and complete an incident form.
    F. Make the case anonymous and discuss it with your colleagues as a learning exercise.

Enter your answer:

1st	
2nd	
3rd	

Suggested answer 3

From this scenario, you should appreciate that a number of issues should be considered:

- Patient safety
- Critical incident event reporting
- Accountability of care
- Avoidance of blame culture and marginalization.

Option A is a very appropriate course of action and should be carried out immediately.

Option B is completely inappropriate because the patient remains at risk with trimethoprim on the drug chart. You would also be ignoring the direct concerns of the pharmacist.

Option C is inappropriate as it is the prescribing doctor's responsibility to ensure drug allergies are checked before prescribing any medication. This is akin to 'passing the buck'.

Option D may be seen as being confrontational. Errors do occur and there should be structured feedback to enable lessons to be learnt from them. However, colleagues should not feel 'on the spot' and this approach is likely to be counterproductive and will not facilitate team work.

Option E in this context is the only other appropriate option. However normally there are hierarchical steps to be taken before escalation to director level (i.e. report the incident to your consultant). If, on the other hand, there is inadequate response from senior members of the team, then escalation is very appropriate especially if patient safety is the focus. Completing a critical incident report would be appropriate and should be seen as a learning exercise to avoid any similar occurrences from happening in the future. Incident forms are not a blaming tool and trainees are expected to participate in the scheme.

Option F is very appropriate and should be seen as a learning exercise to highlight real life medical errors. It gives members of the team a chance to analyse and reflect on their action and modify their future practice.

Therefore the three most appropriate options would be:

1st	A
2nd	F
3rd	E

Question 4

You are an FY2 in general practice. You are called urgently to the reception area where a patient has collapsed and has no pulse. What do you do next?

Choose the three most appropriate actions:

    A. Ask for an urgent ECG.
    B. Ask for an urgent ABG (arterial blood gas).
    C. Call 999.
    D. Start immediate CPR (cardiopulmonary resuscitation).
    E. Give adrenaline IV immediately.
    F. Shout for help from your colleagues.

Enter your answer:

1st	
2nd	
3rd	

Suggested answer 4

This scenario deals with the emergency care of a patient in general practice.

Option A in this scenario is not appropriate. It would create an unnecessary delay in CPR. Some practices may not have an ECG machine anyway.

Option B would be impossible in most general practice surgeries.

Option C is appropriate and must be done urgently. You could delegate this task to the receptionist, while you assess the patient and commence CPR.

Option D is very appropriate. CPR must be commenced immediately. Some GP surgeries have an AED (automated external defibrillator) on site.

Option E is incorrect. Adrenaline is not required immediately in CPR.

Option F is appropriate and you must shout for help immediately as per resuscitation guidelines.

The three most appropriate options would be:

1st	F
2nd	D
3rd	C

Question 5

You are an SHO in hospital. The FY2 doctor on your team tells you that he is addicted to ecstasy. He has been taking it almost every evening following a recent break up with his long-term girlfriend. He is confiding in you for support and asks you not to inform anyone. At present there is no impact on his work or patient safety. What would you do next?

Rank the following in order (1, most appropriate; 4, least appropriate)

A. Tell him you will keep the matter a secret.
B. Ask your registrar's advice.
C. Offer your support, but say he must discuss this issue with the consultant.
D. Inform your consultant if he does not tell them of his addiction because you have no choice.

Enter your answer:

1st	
2nd	
3rd	
4th	

Suggested answer 5

This scenario is difficult and raises many points of the key GMC documents 'Duties of a doctor' and 'Good Medical Practice'.

- Protecting patient safety
- Working with colleagues that best serve patients' interests
- Never discriminate unfairly against colleagues
- Protecting patients from risk posed by another colleague's conduct, performance or health
- Maintaining confidentiality.

Option A is unacceptable because by doing nothing and keeping the matter a secret you place patient safety at risk and this may have detrimental effects on your colleague, and ramifications for you. They are confiding in you and therefore seeking your help: colluding with them will be detrimental – their addiction may spiral out of control and influence both work and social life. In general, you must never collude with a 'dangerous colleague' or any illegal activity.

Option B may seem reasonable action, but you are breaching confidence and your actions could be misconstrued as gossip, which would create friction between team members.

Option C is the most appropriate from the given options because you are encouraging your colleague to open up and seek help for himself while providing support.

Option D is an appropriate action as you will have given your colleague a chance to disclose the information himself. You alone cannot solve all the problems and you will need help from seniors and management to enact the appropriate measures.

Given this information, the most appropriate order would be:

1st	C
2nd	D
3rd	B
4th	A

Question 6

You are a GP and it's Christmas. A patient brings you a box of chocolates and a bottle of red wine. What do you do?

Choose the three most appropriate actions:

A. Explain to the patient that the government does not let doctors accept gifts.
B. Accept the gift thanking the patient and telling him he is very kind.
C. Refuse the gift and admonish the patient for putting you in this situation.
D. Accept the gift and inform your colleagues and practice manager.
E. Accept the gift informing him that he shouldn't have gone out of his way.
F. Request that he makes a donation instead to the whole practice.
G. Contact the GMC.
H. Accept the gift, but suggest that you prefer white wine.

Enter your answer:

1st	
2nd	
3rd	

Suggested answer 6

This is a common scenario involving the following issues:

- Conscience
- Professional integrity
- Probity and honesty
- Maintaining doctor–patient relationships.

Long-standing patients may bring small gifts and this is acceptable. Large monetary gifts are unacceptable and should be politely declined. Charitable donations to the department or practice are allowable if made through the proper channels. If you have any doubt, then it is appropriate to discuss with your colleagues, practice manager and defence union. Any interaction with your patient should be mindful of maintaining the doctor–patient relationship and caution should be taken in case this is disrupted.

Option A is incorrect. Option B is an appropriate action. You are grateful for the gesture and have a positive influence on the doctor–patient relationship.

Option C will adversely affect the doctor–patient relationship. You may have to politely explain why you cannot accept a gift from a patient, particularly if it is a large or expensive gift.

Option D is appropriate, although not compulsory. A practice manager can log all gifts and this can mean open declaration.

Option E is entirely appropriate and gives the impression that you are grateful for his gesture, while expressing that he didn't need to go out of his way.

Option F is unreasonable as he is only making a small Christmas gesture to you. It may well be out of his economic reach to make any donations to the practice.

Option G is inappropriate. If monetary donations were being made you would discuss this with your defence union and may take advice from the GMC.

Option H is clearly inappropriate and nonsensical. You should never solicit gifts from patients.

Given the above the three most appropriate options would be:

1st	B
2nd	E
3rd	D

Question 7

You are an FY2 doctor in general practice. You saw a patient last week who attended with palpitations and you agreed to request an ECG for her. But you forgot to request it and have only just remembered. What do you do next?

Choose two options from:

A. Tell your GP supervisor.
B. Call the patient to check she is okay and inform her the referral was lost in the post.
C. Request the ECG immediately.
D. Do nothing.
E. Call the patient and tell her to attend A&E urgently.
F. Call the cardiology registrar on call for advice.

Enter your answer:

1st
2nd

Suggested answer 7

This scenario highlights professional integrity and the need to be organized during your working practice.

Option A is entirely appropriate: your supervisor is responsible for your training and actions and therefore will need to know of any errors. They will also be able to advise you on alternative ways of rectifying the error.

Option B is dishonest to say it is lost in the post and therefore wrong.

Option C is appropriate because while time has been lost, there is no need for further delays.

Option D is clearly not a feasible option.

Option E would be an inappropriate use of A&E resources. This would be appropriate if the patient was unwell or had an episode of syncope during palpitations.

Option F is reasonable, but ranks lower than options A and C because the error is an administrative one, and therefore they cannot help further.

Therefore, the correct answers are:

1st	A
2nd	C

Question 8

A young Polish-speaking lady attends your morning surgery accompanied by her boyfriend who speaks little English. The boyfriend tells you they had unprotective intercourse and would like the emergency contraceptive pill. She looks anxious but you are unable to talk directly to her. What do you do?

Rank the following in order (1, most appropriate; 5, least appropriate)

A. Ask the boyfriend to interpret the consultation for you.
B. Attempt to communicate with the young girl using diagrams and the odd English word known by her.
C. Arrange for a language line consultation using interpreters over the telephone available 24 hours a day to consult with the girl alone.
D. Arrange for another appointment tomorrow with a booked interpreter.
E. Tell them that you are unable to help, as you cannot understand them.

Enter your answer:

1st	
2nd	
3rd	
4th	
5th	

Suggested answer 8

The key issues are:

- Communication
- Coercion
- Maintaining doctor–patient relationships
- Professional integrity.

A. Option A is not appropriate as the statement suggests that his English is not perfect. Furthermore, we cannot guarantee he will accurately translate the young woman's wishes and we cannot exclude coercion.

B. Option B is unsafe and you are unlikely to achieve any positive workable outcome.

C. Option C is an appropriate and widely accepted means of communication within the health service. In lieu of a physical interpreter, language line is a telephone service that will enable you to have an impartial interpreter. While not perfect, it is a realistic and practical 'work around'.

D. Option D is an appropriate action, but they may not keep the appointment and may seek alternative, less safe options to the emergency pill. Longer delays will also reduce the efficacy of the emergency pill.

E. Option E is unacceptable. There are always means of communicating via language line or prebooked interpreters and alternatives should be sought.

Given this information the most appropriate order would be:

1st	C
2nd	D
3rd	A
4th	B
5th	E

Question 9

You see a newly registered patient. He is a previous heroin addict and is requesting methadone. You do not have any information on the patient other than what he tells you. His notes from his previous practice are yet to arrive. What do you do in this situation?

Choose the two most appropriate actions:

A. Ask the patient to restart his heroin to prevent withdrawal symptoms.
B. Send the patient to A&E.
C. Tell the patient that you cannot prescribe anything until his old notes arrive.
D. Ask him what amount of methadone he has previously been taking and prescribe that amount for 7 days.
E. Speak to the psychiatry SHO on call for advice.
F. Telephone his old GP for further information.
G. Guess an amount that you think is reasonable given his history and prescribe this to him on a daily basis until the notes arrive.

Enter your answer:

1st	
2nd	

Suggested answer 9

This scenario raises issues regarding:

- Management of drug addiction symptoms
- Maintaining doctor–patient relationships
- Professional integrity.

Let us consider each of the options individually.

Option A is clearly unacceptable and you should never encourage risk behaviour which places the patient at significant harm.

Option B is unhelpful: this is not a medical emergency and the A&E will be in no better position to determine the patient's previous methodone use. This simply delays care and wastes resources.

Option C is appropriate, but the patient may not appreciate it! Managing his addiction safely will require his old notes: a too high prescription may lead to overdose or encourage illegal behaviour, such as selling surplus methadone.

Option D is very unsafe and can potentially lead to overdose. Patients with addiction can be unreliable witnesses to their past medical history and drug use.

Option E seems reasonable but, similar to deferring to A&E, will achieve little because they will need the same information that you do to safely prescribe methadone.

Option F is very appropriate. It is very straightforward to contact the previous general practice and get more information about the patient in question. An alternative is contacting the pharmacy the patient attends – the majority have directly observed methadone use in a community pharmacy and they will have records of the amount used.

Option G is very unsafe and should not be done.

Given the above, the two most appropriate options would be:

1st	F
2nd	C

Question 10

You are an FY2 doctor in hospital. Your FY1 has been complaining that he has not been permitted to be involved in patient management decisions or perform procedures. During a peri-arrest situation you ask him to take an arterial blood gas sample for analysis. Instead, he walks away angrily saying this is a task for a healthcare assistant.

Choose the three most appropriate actions:

A. Demand the FY1 returns and admonish him for his disregard for your orders.
B. Once the patient is stabilized, discuss his feelings in an informal manner.
C. Apologise to the FY1 and ask him to 'run' the peri-arrest situation.
D. Take the blood sample for analysis yourself.
E. Once the patient is stabilized, inform your consultant.
F. Call for help from your hospital peri-arrest team.
G. Complain to other FY1 doctors about his behaviour.

Enter your answer:

1st	
2nd	
3rd	

Suggested answer 10

This scenario raises issues regarding:

- Identifying a colleague in difficulty
- Dealing with difficult colleagues
- Prioritizing emergency situations
- Maintaining patient safety.

Look at each option in turn:

While such behaviour may evoke anger in you, option A is not helpful as this will lead to more resentment from the FY1 doctor. Clearly they feel undervalued and are perhaps overwhelmed by their job which manifests in this petulant behaviour. Admonishing them in front of colleagues and an unwell patient is not appropriate.

Option B is clearly an appropriate action. You should explore his feelings and why he thought such behaviour was acceptable. He should be informed that behaviour is dangerous and that he may need remedial measures.

Option C appears to appease him but could be considered to pandering to petulant behaviour. Furthermore, asking a junior colleague to take over a medically serious situation is inappropriate. You may be too inexperienced to safely supervise the FY1 in a peri-arrest situation.

Option D appears to get the task done, but is inappropriate as you may be the only senior doctor present. You should ask another member of the ward team to do this and stay with the patient.

Option E is a correct action once the situation has resolved. The FY1 doctor needs senior guidance and doctors in difficulty need to be recognized and helped early.

Option F is also appropriate because you need an extra pair of hands to treat the unwell patient.

Option G is unproductive and creates disharmony in your place of work. Seniors should be involved rather than gossiping with junior colleagues.

The three appropriate actions would be:

1st	F
2nd	B
3rd	E

Question 11

You are an FY2 doctor in A&E. You are on annual leave and on your way to a restaurant with family. You witness a drunk homeless person who is a frequent A&E attender staggering around. What should you do?

Choose the two most appropriate actions:

A. Call the ambulance service.
B. Do nothing.
C. Ask if he is okay and requires assistance.
D. Forcibly walk him to A&E and then leave.
E. Ask another passer-by to help the man.

Enter your answer:

1st	
2nd	

Suggested answer 11

From the above scenario you may quickly appreciate that a number of issues have arisen:

- Conscience
- Professional integrity

Let us consider each of the options individually.

Option A is inappropriate, there is no apparent emergency and the patient is drunk. You should see if he needs assistance first.

Option B is an acceptable option here. Normally the 'do nothing' option is inappropriate, however, based on the information given, no medical intervention is required. He is drunk and this is likely his status quo.

Option C is the most appropriate action as you are checking to see if he requires assistance and based on his response you can then proceed accordingly. It is likely he is simply drunk and will send you away. You will need to make a rapid assessment of the situation and seek help if necessary.

Option D is reasonable only if he wants help. It will be very counterproductive if you take him against his will and he may cause disruption in the A&E waiting area.

Option E is inappropriate. You are effectively passing on the responsibility to another individual when it is your duty.

Given this information, the most appropriate order would be:

1st	C
2nd	B

Question 12

You are the FY2 doctor on call for medicine. Your supervising registrar is a locum who is unfamiliar with the hospital. He hands you his pager and says he will be back in an hour. Two hours later you are still alone and called to see an anuric patient in acute renal failure with no intravenous access on medical HDU (high dependency unit).

Choose the three most appropriate actions:

A. Call the intensive care department and seek their urgent review of the patient.
B. Refuse to hold the registrar pager and hand it to the clinical nurse manager.
C. Call the medical consultant on-call and inform him of the situation.
D. Start making a formal written complaint about the locum registrar.
E. Ask the nurses to await the return of the locum registrar and leave.
F. Call the clinical nurse manager for help.

Enter your answer:

1st	
2nd	
3rd	

Suggested answer 12

This is a complex scenario which initially appears difficult. The key issue here is identifying your limitations and seeking help.

Option A is entirely appropriate and medically correct based on the information presented. As a junior member of the team you are not expected to manage difficult patients alone and help should be sought early.

Option B is not reasonable. It is a doctor's pager.

Option C is correct and appropriate. The on-call medical consultant is ultimately responsible for the care delivered and would expect to be called during emergencies. He or she may need to come into the hospital to help.

Option D suggests making a complaint which appears to be appropriate but this should be done when the medical situation has been resolved. This could be done the following day. An investigation will be required and the absence of the locum registrar could be entirely innocent – for example, he may be lost in the hospital!

Option E is clearly inappropriate and is not medically safe.

Option F is entirely reasonable: the clinical nurse managers are highly experienced nursing colleagues who may have encountered the situation before and can help with other mundane tasks while you tackle the sick patient.

Therefore the correct options are:

1st	A
2nd	C
3rd	F

Question 13

You are an FY2 on board a flight to the United States. You have had several alcoholic beverages. A flight attendant asks for medical help with a breathless patient.

Rank the following in order:

    A. Attend the unwell passenger urgently.
    B. Ask the pilot to land the plane as an emergency.
    C. Do not declare yourself as a medical doctor.
    D. Declare yourself as a medical doctor, but explain that you have drunk alcohol and therefore have impaired judgement.
    E. Ask the attendant to check if any other healthcare providers are on board.

Enter your answer:

1st	
2nd	
3rd	
4th	
5th	

Suggested answer 13

This is a complex situation of which you may have first-hand experience. In general, flight crews now have access to basic medical supplies and can communicate with a ground team which includes a medical practitioner. However, it is appropriate that a doctor on a flight makes their presence known if it is requested. Your judgement will be impaired in the presence of alcohol and this should be declared at the first opportunity.

Option A is a possible response, however does not acknowledge that you are intoxicated and this should be done first.

Option B is a drastic response which may be required. However, you have not yet assessed the patient and therefore this is less appropriate. There is a considerable cost implication in an emergency landing and a pilot will make a decision together with a medical practitioner on the ground based on a protocol. It is unlikely this decision will rest with you alone – but this can occur with smaller airline companies!

Option C is unacceptable and is a probity issue. You should let the team know you are available even if they decide they do not need you.

Option D is the correct option and should be done as soon as help is requested.

Option E is also correct – often there may be many medical practitioners on a plane.

Considering the above, the correct responses are:

1st	D
2nd	E
3rd	A
4th	B
5th	C

Question 14

You are an FY2 doctor in hospital. The IT department contacts you about accessing adult pornography websites on the doctors' office computers. The logs document the access occurred over a weekend when you were not working.

Choose the three most appropriate actions:

A. Inform the police.
B. Explain that you were not working that weekend and provide evidence to support this.
C. Refuse to participate in the enquiry.
D. Inform your consultant.
E. Blame the locum doctor to whom you gave your computer log-on details.
F. Admonish the IT department for not having stricter website controls.
G. Contact your medical defence union.

Enter your answer:

1st	
2nd	
3rd	

Suggested answer 14

This scenario involves following hospital policies and being responsible for your computer log-on details. This situation can occur if you share your log-on details with others or if you leave a computer logged on.

Let us consider each of the options individually:

Option A is not necessary. Adult pornography is not illegal, although viewing at work will be against hospital policy. You do not have evidence of anybody performing an illegal offence.

Option B is appropriate and you should take action to prove your innocence by co-operating with the enquiry fully. Friends and family who know you were not on hospital site at the time of offence will help.

Option C is inappropriate because it does not help you. While you may think the rota is fairly clear, the IT department and investigating individuals cannot be expected to defend you.

Option D is entirely reasonable and having the support of a senior individual will be important if the case progresses. He or she may need to give a character reference.

Option E is defensive and sets up questions as to why your log-on details were shared: when you were inducted to the hospital, you signed IT policy documents stating you will not share your log-on details.

Option F is confrontational and is likely to anger your accuser!

Option G is reasonable. The defence union will guide you through the appropriate steps and will not be viewed as an admission of guilt.

Given the above, the three most appropriate options would be:

1st	B
2nd	D
3rd	G

Question 15

You are a GP registrar. You see a patient with lower back pain. After examining them, you make a diagnosis of mechanical back pain and suggest a management plan. They are not satisfied and become verbally aggressive. What would you do?

Choose the three most appropriate actions:

A. Retaliate in self-defence and exchange verbal comments.
B. Politely explain to the patient that this is unacceptable behaviour and that they should take a few moments to calm down.
C. Call the police.
D. Leave the room and speak with one of the GP partners.
E. Inform your experienced practice manager of the situation.
F. Inform the primary care trust.
G. Have the patient removed from the practice register.

Enter your answer:

1st	
2nd	
3rd	

Suggested answer 15

This scenario raises issues about maintaining personal safety and the safety of your staff while maintaining professionalism. You must still consider the welfare of the aggressive patient and consider why they are being aggressive.

Let us consider each of the options individually:

Option A is unacceptable and will perpetuate the situation. It is very unprofessional to exchange verbal abuse and you should do everything in your power to calm the situation. If you are physically threatened, you are entitled to proportionate self-defence.

Option B is the most appropriate action. You must maintain control of the situation while giving the patient room for reflection of their actions. Most individuals will realize they are being unreasonable.

Option C based on the scenario above is inappropriate. If the patient was physically abusive or refused to calm down, then involving the police may be reasonable.

Option D is another appropriate action. This again gives the patient time to reflect while removing you from a potentially dangerous situation. Your other GP colleagues will undoubtedly be able to advise you further.

Option E is an appropriate action. Here you are able to call upon the experience and negotiation skills of your practice manager.

Option F is clearly nonsensical: the primary care trust cannot help this acutely aggravated situation.

Option G is inappropriate at this stage. However, this could be considered if the patient had persistent outbursts of abuse towards staff.

Given the above, the three most appropriate options would be:

1st	B
2nd	D
3rd	E

Question 16

You are a GP FY2. A window cleaner attends the surgery and would like a sick note for 3 weeks. He is medically well but wants to attend his daughter's wedding and cannot get time off work. What should you do?

Choose three appropriate actions:

    A. Fabricate an illness and give the patient a sick note.
    B. Admonish the patient for making an illegal request and demand that they leave.
    C. Explain it would be dishonest and therefore you cannot give a sick note.
    D. Ask the patient to explore alternative leave options with his employer.
    E. Discuss if there are any other issues the patient wants to raise.
    F. Suggest he should go to A&E with a fabricated illness.
    G. Ask him to see another GP in the practice.

Enter your answer:

1st	
2nd	
3rd	

Suggested answer 16

This scenario tests whether you will collude with a patient making an inappropriate request and assesses that you will operate within professional boundaries. There is a strong emphasis on reducing the use of sick notes and in particular those issued for dubious medical need.

Option A is clearly wrong and you should not fabricate any illness even if it is to help a patient.

Option B will harm the doctor–patient relationship. He is seeking your help and has perhaps not considered other options to obtain leave from work. This response would prevent him from attending in the future when there is a medical problem.

Option C is appropriate and you should explain that we have a duty to protect the 'sick note' system for only those who medically need it. You should explain this in a positive way such that the patient understands the medical and legal reasons.

Option D is also appropriate as he may not have considered alternative options such as making up leave as overtime another time. You should act as the patient's advocate. You should not contact his employer unless the patient gives clear permission.

Option E is important because patients may in fact be masking true symptoms. It is common for middle-aged men to attend for a seemingly innocuous problem, when they are concerned about something different.

Option F is clearly wrong and is encouraging abuse of the medical system.

Option G would break the patient's confidence in you and suggests that while you may not issue a sick note, somebody else will. This will be inappropriate.

Therefore, the correct options are:

1st	C
2nd	D
3rd	E

Question 17

You are the FY2 in general practice. A 15-year-old girl attends wanting to start the 'pill'. She is having unprotected sex with a 15-year-old boy. She cannot be persuaded to inform her parents and says she will continue to have sex with or without contraception. What would you do?

Choose the two most appropriate actions:

A. Refuse to give her the oral contraceptive pill.
B. Request that she goes home with some information and speaks with her mother.
C. Give her a 1-month's supply of the pill and some condoms, stressing the risk of sexually transmitted infections.
D. Ring her mother during the consultation, informing her of the situation.
E. Discuss the case with a senior member of the team.
F. Ask her to attend the family planning clinic.

Enter your answer:

1st	
2nd	

Suggested answer 17

This scenario involves detailed knowledge of Fraser and Gillick competence. This is also covered later in the book.

Option A is unacceptable as you run the risk of this young girl falling pregnant because she is sexually active.

Option B at first glance seems reasonable, but again the action involves sending the young girl away without the contraception requested. It also raises the question of confidentiality. Perhaps she has not told her parents that she is sexually active. There is again a risk of pregnancy.

Option C is an appropriate action as you are providing her with contraception and reducing the risk of sexually transmitted infections. Normally, the first prescription for the pill will be for 3 months. However, this option is not given here. You should attempt to keep her engaged with the services and provide further education.

Option D is inappropriate as you may be going against her wishes and this will impact on the doctor–patient relationship.

Option E is an appropriate action as you can take advice from a senior member with experience.

Option F may seem reasonable but she may not attend, again raising the risk of pregnancy.

Given the above, the two most appropriate options would be:

1st	C
2nd	E

Question 18

You are the FY2 on a busy general medical ward. You are about to start a consultant ward round. A nurse informs you that a relative of a terminally ill patient would like to speak with you. What would you subsequently do?

Rank the following in order (1, most appropriate; 5, least appropriate):

A. Inform the nurse that you are too busy to see the relative.
B. See the relative immediately.
C. Before the ward round starts, ask the consultant to be excused allowing your house officer to continue on the round.
D. Ask the nurse to speak with the relative to gather more information.
E. Apologise to the relatives in person and arrange a meeting later in the afternoon.

Enter your answer:

1st	
2nd	
3rd	
4th	
5th	

Suggested answer 18

This is a common scenario on busy wards and requires us to manage time appropriately. The patient is terminally ill and the family are likely to have many questions. Recognizing this is essential and will help you answer this question.

Option A is inappropriate and dismissive of the relative. It is unfair on them.

Option B immediately seems to be the most appropriate. However, we must be aware of our commitment to the ward round which will be disrupted by your unexpected absence. Furthermore, you may be called out of your discussion with the family which would be unsatisfactory for all involved. Therefore, the alternative option C would rank higher than option B. Option C also potentially allows the consultant to become involved in the discussion with relatives.

Option D may seem reasonable, but the relatives have specifically asked to speak with a doctor.

Option E is an entirely sensible plan of action. You acknowledge the relative in person and negotiate a time that suits both parties. The ward round can therefore continue with all team members present.

Given this information, the most appropriate order would be:

1st	C
2nd	E
3rd	B
4th	D
5th	A

Question 19

You are FY2 on a medical ward round. Your consultant humiliates the FY1 doctor at the bedside for failing to interpret the patient's ECG. You feel that this was unfair as it was a difficult ECG. What would you do?

Choose the three most appropriate actions:

A. Ask to have a word with the consultant on the ward and express your concerns.
B. Do nothing.
C. Ask the ward sister to speak with the consultant.
D. Contact the clinical director.
E. Ask the consultant to arrange an ECG teaching tutorial.
F. Speak with your FY1 and encourage them to express their concerns about the incident to the consultant.
G. Encourage your house officer to contact the British Medical Association.

Enter your answer:

1st	
2nd	
3rd	

Suggested answer 19

While routine 'teaching by humiliation' has become infrequent, there are still occasions. While some view it constructively, it is inappropriate behaviour on the ward and in front of a patient. It can be viewed as harassment or bullying. We have duty to our colleagues to stop this from happening if we witness it.

Option A is appropriate. The consultant may not recognize that the ECG was difficult and fails to understand that his actions towards the FY1 were inappropriate.

Option B is inappropriate if you witness bullying. Being part of a team means being involved in all aspects of it, including doing things that may be uncomfortable. By doing nothing you collude with the inappropriate behaviour.

Option C is inappropriate because you are passing the buck.

Option D is premature: resolution at a ward level is required. The clinical director would be required if the consultant fails to respond having been informed and other consultant colleagues cannot persuade him that his behaviour is incorrect.

Option E is an elegant solution which will permit training and will allow the consultant to establish what level of knowledge there is among the junior doctors. This will hopefully prevent future outbursts.

Option F is appropriate. The FY1 is at the centre of the incident and of the subsequent complaint. The discussion may have more effect on the consultant if initiated by the house officer.

Option G is inappropriate at this stage. However, if there were no local resolution of the situation then you could consider this an appropriate action.

Given the above, the three most appropriate options would be:

1st	A
2nd	E
3rd	F

Question 20

You are the on-call duty GP requested to go on a home visit for a patient with known COPD. Before entering the patient's home, you are confronted with an aggressive relative demanding hospital admission for the patient. You have not seen or assessed the patient yet. What do you do?

Choose the three most appropriate actions:

    A. Refuse to see the patient and return back to the practice.
    B. Call the ambulance.
    C. Contact the police.
    D. Appreciate the relative's concerns and request that you are allowed to examine the patient to make this decision.
    E. Call the practice for support from another GP.
    F. Confront the relative.
    G. Ask to speak to the patient to understand their views.

Enter your answer:

1st	
2nd	
3rd	

Suggested answer 20

In this scenario you should consider both personal and patient safety. Home visits can involve an element of 'going into the unknown'.

Option A is unacceptable because you have not been able to assess the patient and make a safe clinical decision.

Option B may be appropriate especially if you are unable to gain access to the patient. The relative may allow paramedic assessment as it gives an impression of possible hospital admission. Some may consider this a waste of resources, but if not resolved now, the relatives are likely to call for an ambulance.

Option C is inappropriate at this stage. However, if there were physical aggression then you would appropriately consider this action.

Option D is the most appropriate action as you are trying to alleviate the relatives concerns, while attempting to gain access to assess the patient.

Option E is inappropriate as another member of the practice is unlikely to reverse the current situation as the relative is demanding hospital admission.

Option F is unacceptable. You should never aggravate the situation but try to calm it.

Option G is appropriate. The source of tension may stem from the patient not wanting hospital admission and the relative trying to ensure this happens.

Given the above, the three most appropriate options would be:

1st	D
2nd	G
3rd	B

Question 21

You are an FY2 in a busy general practice surgery. You see a 2-year-old girl with her mother who has a suspected chest infection when you notice some suspicious scalds to both her lower legs. What would you do next?

Rank the following in order (1, most appropriate; 5, least appropriate):

A. Speak to your colleagues who have seen the child before.
B. Take no action on the scalds and just deal with the chest infection.
C. Speak to the police.
D. Contact the local child protection officer.
E. Ask the mother about the scalds.

Enter your answer:

1st	
2nd	
3rd	
4th	
5th	

Suggested answer 21

Child protection issues are critical and must be at the forefront of your mind when dealing with children. You must be cautious not to jump to conclusions without prior explanation.

Option A is a wholly appropriate action. Your colleagues should be able to shed some light on to the dynamics of the household and whether the colleagues share any of your concerns. Ideally, this should have already been documented in the medical notes.

Option B is inappropriate. Having noted the leg scalds, you are duty bound to investigate as you are not aware of how they happened. You cannot guarantee that the child will be safe without further enquiry.

Option C may be an appropriate action, however you would explore the circumstances on a local level first and then escalate to the police if needed.

Option D is an appropriate action as they may have further records where concerns have been raised regarding the physical and mental health of the child. If there are no previous records, then this episode can be documented.

Option E would be the most appropriate action as you are giving the mother a chance to explain the situation and can observe her response. Experience is required in managing these cases.

Given this information, the most appropriate order would be:

1st	E
2nd	A
3rd	D
4th	C
5th	B

Question 22

You are a GP registrar on a home visit to a nursing home. Your patient is elderly and tells you that the care home staff deliberately try to hurt him. What would you do next?

Rank the following in order (1, most appropriate; 5, least appropriate):

A. Dismiss him as being a little bit senile.
B. Discuss your concerns with the care home manager.
C. Demand an explanation from the team leader.
D. Try to gather more specific information from the patient.
E. Inform your GP trainer.

Enter your answer:

1st	
2nd	
3rd	
4th	
5th	

Suggested answer 22

Patient safety and vulnerable adults should be considered in this scenario.

Option A is very inappropriate, and you should take all allegations by a vulnerable adult seriously: you cannot leave him in a potentially dangerous situation.

Option B is an appropriate action. The care home manager should be made aware of any issues especially those involving claims of neglect and inappropriate treatment. The manager can then launch his or her own enquiry into the events.

Option C is very confrontational because you are 'demanding' an explanation. It would be appropriate if it were phrased tactfully and in a non-threatening manner.

Option D is the most appropriate action as you must clarify the situation and understand precisely what is happening before further action can be taken.

Option E is an appropriate action as you will be able to utilize the experience of your trainer.

Given this information, the most appropriate order would be:

1st	D
2nd	B
3rd	E
4th	C
5th	A

Question 23

You are the FY2 in general practice. You review a patient with poorly controlled epilepsy with recurrent seizures. His wife is present and tells you he is still driving despite you previously informing him that he should cease to drive and inform the DVLA. What would you do?

Choose the three most appropriate actions:

A. Educate him of the dangers of continuing to drive.
B. Inform him that you are going to inform the DVLA and then do so.
C. Ask the patient to voluntarily inform the DVLA and cease to drive.
D. Contact the police.
E. Pursue the issue no further, you have done your best.
F. Ask his wife to persuade him.

Enter your answer:

1st	
2nd	
3rd	

Suggested answer 23

Epilepsy, recent TIAs and diabetics requiring insulin driving heavy goods vehicles or public service vehicles are common questions.

Here, the common variant of uncontrolled epilepsy is considered. Patients should not drive for 1 year since the last fit. If patients continue to drive despite warning, doctors can inform the DVLA. This breach of confidentiality is in the interests of public safety and you must inform the patient that you are going to do this.

Option A is appropriate as the patient may not be aware of the possibility of further seizures while continuing to drive.

Option B is appropriate if the patient persisted not to inform the DVLA himself. Therefore, this option would rank below option C.

Option C is appropriate because the patient may have forgotten the original discussion regarding driving when his epilepsy was first diagnosed.

Option D is inappropriate at this stage. If, however, he refused to cease driving then this could be considered.

Option E is clearly inappropriate as there is potential for the patient to have a seizure while driving, posing significant risk to the public.

Option F, while not entirely incorrect, is less favourable than the other options.

Given the above, the three most appropriate options would be:

1st	A
2nd	C
3rd	B

Question 24

You are the FY2 in general practice. Before the start of his morning surgery, you notice the GP partner is intoxicated. What would you do?

Rank the following in order (1, most appropriate; 5, least appropriate)

A. Inform the GP partner that you are concerned that he is intoxicated and ask him to go home.
B. Confront the GP partner and demand an explanation.
C. Allow him to see patients and speak to him after lunch when he is more sober.
D. Speak to the GP principal of your concerns and ask them to cover the surgery.
E. Tell the patients that the GP partner is unwell and unable to attend his surgery today.

Enter your answer:

1st	
2nd	
3rd	
4th	
5th	

Suggested answer 24

Patient safety and ensuring your colleagues are safe to practice are key issues in this scenario. This is a common scenario in interviews and exams.

Option A is an appropriate first action. The GP partner should realize that he is intoxicated and that his judgement will be impaired. He should agree to go home. Difficulties will arise if he ignores you.

Option B suggests confrontation which will not help a potentially delicate situation. As the more junior colleague you will need tact.

Option C is clearly a wholly inappropriate action, as patient safety will be compromised.

Option D is an essential. The most senior GP in the surgery should be aware of what is happening and should cover patients who no longer have a doctor to see them!

Option E is important because some patients may prefer to come back another day and this may ease the pressure on the remaining doctors covering.

Here, the options appear difficult to organize, but clearly the intoxicated GP must be removed first, then cover sought to replace him. Informing patients then takes the next priority. Confrontation is always to be avoided and therefore ranks lowly. Allowing him to continue surgery while intoxicated is clearly dangerous and therefore this ranks last.

1st	A
2nd	D
3rd	E
4th	B
5th	C

Question 25

You are the FY2 in general practice. Your patient makes several abusive and racist comments directed towards you. What would you do?

Rank the following in order (1, most appropriate; 5, least appropriate):

    A. Continue trying to see the patient, explaining that you are trying to help.
    B. Ask the patient to leave.
    C. Have the patient removed from the practice list.
    D. Ask for help from your GP trainer.
    E. Confront the patient and request that they stop.

Enter your answer:

1st	
2nd	
3rd	
4th	
5th	

Suggested answer 25

Difficult patients are unfortunately part and parcel of working in health care. Despite our feelings, we must not discriminate against them and only consider their health as our primary motivating factor in treating them.

Option A is reasonable, although it places you at ongoing risk and you are likely to receive more racist comments.

Option B is an appropriate action and you are perfectly within your rights to ask the patient to leave if they are inappropriate. This situation has the potential to become confrontational if not handled delicately.

Option C is inappropriate at this stage, however should be considered if the patient continues to be abusive to staff. If physical assault were a feature of the above scenario then it would be highly appropriate.

Option D is an appropriate action because this removes you from a potentially unstable situation. Your GP trainer will be able to support you and perhaps deflate the situation. For this reason, this option ranks above option A.

Option E is highly inappropriate and will only perpetuate the situation.

It would be reasonable to try and deflate the situation by seeking your GP trainer who may know the patient well. If the trainer is unavailable, you could try to pacify the patient yourself, but if the patient continues to be abusive, the next option would be to ask the patient to leave. Removing patients from the list is a difficult and long process that is done at the last resort. Confrontation should always be avoided. Therefore, the appropriate order should be:

1st	D
2nd	A
3rd	B
4th	C
5th	E

Question 26

You are the FY2 doctor on medical nights. You assess a patient with decompensated alcoholic liver disease who needs admission. He is refusing admission to the medical assessment unit (MAU) and will only go straight to the gastroenterology ward that is currently full. What would you do?

Rank the following in order (1, most appropriate; 5, least appropriate):

A. Tell him he has no choice.
B. Section him using the Mental Health Act.
C. Admit him directly to the gastroenterology ward, moving a stable patient out.
D. Explain that he needs admitting to MAU for close observation and explore his reasons for not wanting this.
E. Discuss the situation with your senior.

Enter your answer:

1st	
2nd	
3rd	
4th	
5th	

Suggested answer 26

In this scenario, you should recognize that patients with decompensated liver disease have impaired cognitive function. We must make decisions to ensure their safety.

Option A is likely to aggravate the patient and make a difficult situation worse. This should be done cautiously.

Option B is inappropriate at present. We do not have enough information about the patient's cognitive state. The Mental Health Act is not normally employed in patients confused due to organic reasons.

Option C may seem an appropriate action, however, acutely ill patients cannot be monitored closely and there may be less medical support overnight. It is also unfair to have to move a patient during the middle of the night.

Option D is an appropriate action. Here you are exploring his reluctance and may be able to alleviate any misconceptions that he may have. This is also the safest place for him to be monitored.

Option E is an appropriate action, as you can utilize the experience of your senior.

Given this information, the most appropriate order would be:

1st	D
2nd	E
3rd	C
4th	A
5th	B

Question 27

You are a GP registrar seeing a patient who has produced a long list of problems to discuss. You are conscious that you will end up running late if you try to address them all. What would you do?

Choose the three most appropriate actions:

A. Choose the first problem on the list and address this only.
B. Look at the list and ask which are the problems troubling the patient most.
C. Attempt to address each problem and risk running late.
D. Tell the patient to return another day with a double appointment.
E. Give the patient 10 minutes and then stop wherever you are in the consultation.
F. Make an assessment of the listed problems and identify the ones you consider important.

Enter your answer:

1st	
2nd	
3rd	

Suggested answer 27

Patients have complex problems and prioritization is essential in general practice. Empowering patients is also important so they have say in their health care.

Option A is weak because it allows only the discussion of one problem. This may not be the patient's immediate concern leading to them being unhappy with the consultation.

Option B is sensible because control is given to the patient. The onus is on the patient to prioritize their concerns.

Option C may in some instances be considered appropriate. Patients may place equal importance on all problems and feel unsatisfied if these are not addressed. You may have a patient who infrequently attends and may be put off the idea of consulting in the future. However, boundaries may need to be placed if some patients do this repeatedly, delaying the clinic.

Option D is weak because you are not helping them today. The patient may have had to arrange time away from work to attend.

Option E is clearly a weak answer. Potentially none of the problems will be addressed satisfactorily and you risk important ones being forgotten.

Option F is prudent because you can utilize your experience and determine the important problems that need addressing as a priority. Non-life threatening problems can then be deferred. However, the patient may not appreciate this.

Given the above, the three most appropriate options would be:

1st	B
2nd	F
3rd	C

Question 28

A 35-year-old male says chronic neck pain is preventing him sleeping. A colleague gave him a month's prescription for temazepam 1 week previously. He states that he did not have this prescription dispensed and would like zopiclone. What would you do?

Choose the three most appropriate actions:

A. Give him a 1-month supply of zopiclone.
B. Refuse to give him any further sedatives.
C. Issue him with a 7 days of zopiclone and review in 1 week.
D. Set a message alert on the medication page to alert colleagues of this situation.
E. Discuss alternative options that may include trial of amitriptyline.
F. Prescribe him some further temazepam.

Enter your answer:

1st	
2nd	
3rd	

Suggested answer 28

Identifying drug-seeking behaviour is important, but this can be difficult when patients attend different practitioners.

Option A is an inappropriate action, as you cannot account for the previous temazepam prescription. There is room for prescription abuse and the patient may well be back to see another colleague requesting further sedatives.

Option B may be an appropriate action, however the patient may be telling the truth and therefore this could impact on the doctor–patient relationship.

Option C is an appropriate action, as you are taking control of the situation and placing conditions on the prescription. This action will allow you to closely review the patient and hopefully eliminate the potential for abuse.

Option D is an appropriate action. This will allow you to message-prompt your colleagues and alert them to the patient's actions.

Option E is an appropriate action as the patient may not be aware of alternatives to help his chronic pain.

Option F is a poor answer, because there is potential for abuse of the prescription.

Therefore, the most appropriate answer would be:

1st	C
2nd	E
3rd	D

Question 29

You are the on-call GP during a morning surgery. A middle-aged man comes in and demands an x-ray of his right hand which he injured 4 weeks previously. You assess him and believe that this is inappropriate. What would you subsequently do?

Rank the following in order (1, most appropriate; 5, least appropriate):

A. Reassure the patient that you believe his hand is OK and that there is no clinical indication.
B. Point blank refuse the x-ray.
C. Agree to perform the x-ray if he continues to demand one.
D. Ask the patient to see your colleague another day.
E. Explore his reasons for wanting an x-ray.

Enter your answer:

1st	
2nd	
3rd	
4th	
5th	

Suggested answer 29

Here, patient education is essential to prevent unnecessary testing.

Option A is an appropriate action as there is no clinical indication for the x-ray. This should be done in a reassuring manner so the patient is not disappointed with the consultation.

Option B is likely to result in a disgruntled patient.

Option C could be seen as undermining your judgement, but if the result is normal the patient will hopefully respect your clinical acumen. A better alternative would be to agree to do one if symptoms persist rather than simply because the patient continues to demand one!

Option D is inappropriate, as you will simply be passing on the patient to a colleague without dealing with their concerns.

Option E is the most appropriate action as you are exploring the patient's ideas and concerns. Once identified you may be able to alleviate these through subsequent discussion.

Given this information, the most appropriate order would be:

1st	E
2nd	A
3rd	C
4th	B
5th	D

Question 30

You are the FY2 in obstetrics and gynaecology. A nurse pages you to say she has made a drug error and given a dose of low molecular weight heparin twice within an hour. What would you do next?

Choose the three most appropriate actions:

    A. Thank the nurse for telling you and return to the canteen.
    B. Document the sequence of events in the patient's notes.
    C. Ask the nurse to inform the doctor on the next shift.
    D. Thank the nurse for telling you and review the patient.
    E. Tell the nurse you will ensure she is removed from the nursing register.
    F. Explain to the patient what has happened.

Enter your answer:

1st	
2nd	
3rd	

Suggested answer 30

The key components being assessed here are patient safety, learning from mistakes and ensuring there is a 'no blame' culture.

Option A suggests that you would not review the patient and therefore would not be appropriate patient management.

Option B is correct because it emphasizes the importance of documenting errors at the time that they occur. This facilitates root-cause analysis when this drug error is studied in detail later. Completing an incident form would also be appropriate.

Option C is not helpful as you are 'passing the buck'. The scenario does not suggest you are nearing the end of your shift.

Option D is correct and appropriate. The scenario does not give any clinical details about the patient or the clinical implications of having too much low molecular weight heparin. The dose is not given. However, it is entirely appropriate that patient safety is ensured by reviewing the patient and assessing for any harm.

Option E is confrontation and unnecessarily aggressive. You would be surprised that this statement does occasionally happen in reality! You should engender a 'no blame' culture. Clearly an error has occurred but we should consider what led to it. For example, there may be only one nurse trying to manage the entire drug round while dealing with difficult patients.

Option F is also entirely correct. Even if no harm comes to the patient, it is their right to know what happened. Most will not make a formal complaint if they know what happened and that steps are being taken to avoid it from occurring again. A simple apology is important and not an admission of guilt.

Given this information, the most appropriate order would be:

1st	D
2nd	B
3rd	F

SECTION F

Stage 3: Selection centre assessment

Well done for making it to stage 3!

But, there is no time to relax just yet because the crucial stage 3 selection centre is your next hurdle before the home straight. There is little time to prepare for the stage 3 selection centre once the stage 2 results come out. This section will cover details of each part of the stage 3 selection centre and give you tips to help get you through.

There are numerous practice examples in the following chapters. Use these as practise scenarios to help you engage in role-play, prioritization or group exercises with colleagues or in front of the mirror. The examples given are not exhaustive, but should be used to stimulate your thinking and allow you to practise and learn how you could demonstrate your skills. There is no exact way of how to say particular phrases or prioritize certain tasks. You should develop a pattern which is comfortable for you. Incorporate the ideas given in the examples with your experience and personal traits to make them your own.

Remember, irrespective of which specialty you are currently doing, you can practise your skills through your day-to-day interaction with patients and colleagues. Even if you are simply going to take bloods on a patient, try being a little more engaging and practise building a rapport or using particular phrases. Gradually you find it becomes more natural to you (and the task of taking blood becomes more rewarding!).

10 Introduction to the selection centre assessment

Jasdeep Gill

Format of the selection centre

The stage 3 selection centre consists of two assessments: the simulation exercise and written prioritization exercise. Each assessment tests various parts of the GP NPS and it is important that you pass each assessment. It replaces the artificial interview situation in which it can be difficult for applicants to demonstrate their skills and potential.

The simulation exercise involves three role-play activities with you as the doctor and an actor as the patient or colleague. Your role could be in a hospital or GP setting.

The written prioritization exercise involves ranking a series of options in response to a clinical scenario and justifying your ranking. It also requires you to demonstrate reflective practice.

Checklist of things to remember to take with you

There are several things you must remember to take with you to the stage 3 selection centre. If not, you may not be allowed to undertake stage 3. Take the originals and photocopies, because the deanery will want copies for their reference. Prepare two small folders of all your documents and things to remember. In one folder have all the originals to show, and in the other have photocopies with your applicant number clearly marked so that you can leave it with them. However, remember not to misplace or leave behind any originals as it can be difficult and expensive to replace things. Having two folders will simplify things for you on a stressful day.

You will need:

- your applicant number

- originals of photographic identification and proof of address, such as your passport or driving licence

- UK/EEA applicants should take your passport, birth certificate or naturalization papers. Non-UK/EEA applicants must take evidence of your current immigration status and eligibility to work in the UK.

- your medical degree certificate and other qualifications listed in your stage 1 application

- your GMC certificate

- proof of English language proficiency if your undergraduate training was not in English

- all three of your completed and signed clinical references

- your driving licence as proof of driving

- evidence of your foundation competencies if already achieved, or your VTR2 or ARCP forms

- a wrist watch – you will need this in all three exercises. Practise looking discreetly at how much time you have left.

What to expect on the day

Good preparation will go a long way on the day to help you feel less nervous. The venue is likely to be a renowned hotel or conference centre. Plan your journey in advance. If driving, plan for traffic and beware of parking restrictions. If travelling by public transport, find out about any planned works and be prepared in case unexpected delays occur. You should aim to arrive in good time, approximately 30 minutes to an hour beforehand to allow yourself to acclimatize to the venue and feel calm.

Nationally, each selection centre will be conducted slightly differently. But generally the format will involve going through a registration process at which point all your documents, certificates, and references will be verified and checked. You will be given a code or number to divide you into circuits so that everyone rotates round for each exercise.

There will be a short break in between the exercises, which allows time for a breather and a quick coffee. Some applicants find these breaks difficult because sometimes other applicants begin to 'compare' how it went. It is advised not to discuss your exercise or case. If your last exercise went particularly badly, or even well, you should use the break to put it out of your mind. You don't want to go into the next exercise either overly confident or down, because both can negatively impact your performance. Prepare yourself mentally for the next exercise, be positive and ready to give the next exercise your best shot.

Once you have made it through all the exercises at the selection centre, you will be asked to provide some feedback. You will be reminded not to disclose your cases to others. This is particularly important because you are unlikely to be doing anyone a favour. The scenarios are frequently changed or subtly tweaked, which means your case may sound similar, but be completely different in outcome.

Practise, practise, practise … and practise some more!

- The key ingredient to doing well in the stage 3 selection centre is to practise. This will make you a better and well-rounded applicant.

- The GPST national recruitment process is robust and well designed. However, no system is entirely perfect. Sometimes, even the most well-rounded and patient-centred doctor could fall short in the assessment if they fail to practise the tasks being assessed. Do not let this be you!

- Use the examples in this book and your day-to-day consultations and experiences to practise. You should develop and hone your skills so that you are slick and well prepared for the big day.

- Ask another colleague to help you practise. They can be any specialty, but should ideally be good at role-playing as a patient.

11 Simulation exercise

Jasdeep Gill and Rajesh Kumar

Basis and format of the simulation exercise

The consultation is at the heart of general practice. It is the foundation of the doctor–patient relationship. As a GP, the consultation will be your key tool and all else will arise from it. Therefore, the simulation exercise strives to assess your ability to perform in a consultation.

You are likely to be familiar with role-play consultations from your medical school training. A simulated consultation is essential when assessing any doctor, particularly a potential GP. Although this is a simulated consultation, you should treat it as a real-life consultation and imagine yourself with a real patient or colleague. The actors are highly skilled and will display an array of emotions which you should be able to respond to appropriately. The actors are primed to direct the consultation to ensure you are fully assessed. Some people say they would prefer real patients, but the inherent variability of patients will render the exercise less fair. The simulation exercise tests your skills in relation to all parts of the GP NPS:

Clinical knowledge: simulation exercise

Your clinical skills will only be assessed to a small degree. For example, you may be given the diagnosis and have to plan subsequent management or have awareness of how a diagnosis could impact on a patient's life. Do not get flustered if you do not know the exact treatment or management. Remember, you should not bluff your way through it. So you should honestly admit that you do not know something. You should explain to the patient that you will have to find out or discuss with your seniors about a particular aspect and you will contact the patient.

Empathy and sensitivity: simulation exercise

You should consider the patient as the central focus of care. For this exercise, you should ensure the environment and atmosphere is suitable for the patient and the context of the scenario. For example, if the brief highlights that the patient is a recent widow who has come to see you to complain about the death of her husband, then it would be inappropriate for you to be upbeat and jovial. Instead, you should display empathy and sensitivity by appearing warm, inviting, sincere and expressing your condolences. Your tone of voice will need to respond to the scenario and will need to change according to the patient's reactions.

You should always explore the role-player's perspective, particularly on their diagnosis, lifestyle and management plan. Acknowledge their fears and emotions. Do not make them feel hurried or pressured, and allow the role-player time to open up to you.

Communication skills: simulation exercise

You must display effective patient interaction and communication skills via role play. Effective communication is multifactorial and relates to your ability to:

- Adjust appropriately to verbal and non-verbal cues.
- Listen actively.
- Ask plenty of open and appropriate closed questions to gather information.
- Use non-medical jargon.
- Adapt your language, behaviour and skills to suit the situation or patient.

- Explore the role-player's ideas, concerns and expectations.
- Explain things with clarity.
- Check the role-player's understanding of what they know and what you have told them.
- Summarize for the role-player and safety net.
- Offer patient information leaflets or resources which may help the role-player, if appropriate.

You are likely to have at least a couple of years' experience with patient consultations. Next time you are in a consultation, run through the above pointers to help structure your consultation and aid your communication skills. Remember, it's like a driving test – be overt with your communication skills so the examiner sees and can give you marks. For example, display active listening by mirroring the patient, nodding and using simple encouragement like 'and then …?'

Conceptual thinking and problem solving: simulation exercise

The art of history taking and diagnosing a condition in itself involves conceptual thinking. You would have to display these skills during this exercise and then construct a joint management plan involving the role-player. There is no such thing as 'one size fits all', so you will need to think of a solution and tailor your plan to suit the situation. You will need to use open and some closed questions to help you analyse possible patterns or underlying issues and identify potential different diagnoses.

Coping with pressure: simulation exercise

You may have to demonstrate your ability to cope with pressure via 'difficult' or 'challenging' consultations. These could range from an angry patient who wishes to make a complaint to a bereaved widow who wants to end her life.

You should keep calm throughout the consultation. Depending on the nature of the scenario, you must also display the appropriate communication skills to correctly handle the role-player's emotions and explore their concerns or expectations. It is important for you to appear flexible and to reach an agreed management plan with the role-player. When coping with pressure, you should always maintain perspective on the overall situation. This could involve maintaining a holistic approach when dealing with an angry patient.

Organization and planning: simulation exercise

This exercise will assess your organizing and planning skills through several means. Your overall consultation should be organized and have clear structure. You should use sign-posting to structure the consultation and make it clear to the patient and examiner where you are going with your questions. Use regular summaries to confirm with the patient that you have got it right so far and to demonstrate to the examiner that you are actively absorbing and processing the information. Again, like a driving test, make your skills outwardly obvious.

Your ability to ascertain and prioritize the role-player's agenda could be assessed. Depending on the nature of your scenario, your patient could have a 'shopping list' of issues and you may have to negotiate with them to discuss the most pressing issues first and plan for another consultation if needed for any remaining issues. But remember that the issues that concern you as the doctor may not correspond to those most concerning the patient.

For example, if an elderly patient comes to you with three issues: pain from chronic arthritis which limits her daily, one episode of sudden visual loss which lasted few seconds and needing a flu jab. Which would you prioritize first? But which is the patient more likely to find most bothersome? Chances are the patient would be more interested in resolving her daily pain from arthritis, but you would be interested in finding out more about the episode of visual loss which could be amarousis fugax. You may be able to cover these two issues in one consultation, and then explain that the flu jab could be given by the nurse. This may not be ideal, but at least you are managing all of the patient's issues and using colleagues to help you. This is a practical solution which demonstrates you know the realities of life.

Managing others and team involvement: simulation exercise

Having awareness of the multidisciplinary team and appropriate community orientation is helpful for this exercise. For example, if your scenario involves a teacher with a diagnosis of multiple sclerosis, then you should highlight the need for specialist involvement, multiple sclerosis speciality nurses, physiotherapists, continence advisers, speech therapists and the potential need to liaise with her employer to address occupational issues.

Professional integrity: simulation exercise

As a professional, you must demonstrate respect for your patient and colleagues. You must also be accountable and accept responsibility for your actions. For example, if you find yourself in a challenging consultation with a patient who wants to complain about your colleague, you must apologise to the patient and not apportion blame or disrespect your colleague. You will not be able to show yourself in a good light, by degrading a colleague. Your comments may also have a negative affect on the patient's trust within the system.

The scenario may require you to act within professional boundaries and be aware of your personal limitations. For example, a patient who is banned from driving due to a medical condition may push you to say that they are allowed to drive.

Learning and personal development: simulation exercise

As GPs or 'generalists' it is difficult to know everything about everything. We can manage this by recognizing and addressing the gaps in our knowledge. These gaps are often identified in practice during consultations or when we reflect on the consultation afterwards. If there was something during the consultation that you could not answer then this is an unmet patient need and a doctor's educational need. These are often referred to as 'PUN' (patient's unmet need) and 'DEN' (doctor's educational need). If not already, it should definitely become an important part of your continued learning as a doctor.

Example marking scheme

The role-player will feedback to the examiner about how you made him or her feel and your skills in relation to the GP NPS from the patient's perspective. These comments may be used to inform your assessment for this exercise.

Use the example mark scheme while you practise. Ask your colleagues to mark your consultation. Use it to guide your development and identify areas you need to focus on.

What to expect on the day

The exact format of this exercise will vary between deaneries. You will be directed to the room where your simulated consultation will take place. Often this is a hotel bedroom or small conference room. Do not be put off by other furniture in the room. However, you should be seen to check that the chairs are arranged adequately. The diagrams in Figure 11.1 indicate different arrangements for a consultation.

Being seated face to face, particularly with a desk in between you and a patient, can be considered as confrontational and may be intimidating. Sitting at the corner of a table is more acceptable, for example at an angle of approximately 90–150° between the doctor and patient, because it is considered more open and inviting while allowing both the patient and doctor to feel comfortable in their personal space.

Where possible you should avoid any barriers between you and a patient, such as a desk or paperwork. However, it may not be physically possible to rearrange fixed furniture in a hotel or conference room. In such situations, you should at least demonstrate to the examiner how you would like to rearrange the layout. You are not expected to physically examine the patient, so do not be put off if there is a bed in the room.

Table 11.1 Example mark scheme

		Insufficient evidence	Needs further development	Satisfactory	Competent
Empathy and sensitivity	Creates suitable environment				
	Explores patient's concerns, expectations and perspective				
	Acknowledges patient's feelings and emotions				
	Patient as central focus of care				
Communication skills	Builds rapport with role-player				
	Uses suitable open and closed questions				
	Active listening and non-verbal communication				
	Uses appropriate language				
	Summarizes and 'sign posts' during consultation				
Conceptual thinking and problem solving	Identify and address the problem				
	Think of and negotiate solutions to the problem				
	Is analytical and flexible				
Coping with pressure	Identify stressful or challenging circumstances				
	Display coping mechanisms				
	Identify own limitations and when to seek help				
Organization and planning	Prioritizes issues appropriately				
	Constructs a clear and shared management plan				
	Completes consultation within given time				
Managing others and teams	Able to manage difficult situations				
	Appropriate use of multidisciplinary team				
Professional integrity	Demonstrates respect for patient and peers				
	Operates within professional boundaries				
	Takes responsibility for actions				
	Is honest				
Learning and personal development	Identifies gaps in knowledge or experience				
	Motivated to learn and update knowledge				
Clinical skills	Excludes 'red flags'				
	Appropriate safety netting				

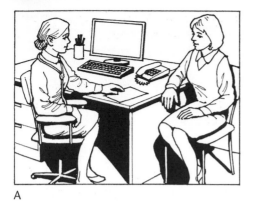

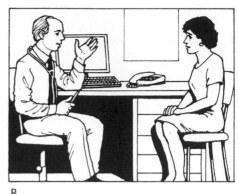

A   B

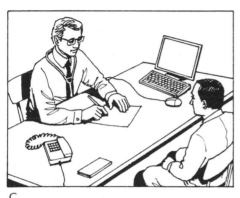

Figure 11.1 Examples of doctor–patient seating configurations.
A) Seated at corner of desk – acceptable.
B) Seated by corner of desk – acceptable.
C) Seated opposite with barrier – not acceptable.

C

You will meet the examiner who will confirm who you are and your applicant number. Remember the assessment starts from the moment you meet the examiner. The examiners are often GPs or hospital consultants and will have been through specific training to undertake this assessment. The examiner will give you a 'doctor's brief' to read which contains information about the scenario. You will have about 5 minutes to read the brief and clarify with the examiner if you have any questions.

The examiner should confirm how long you have for this exercise. It can vary between some deaneries, but for the majority there will be 20 minutes to complete this exercise. You do not have to use the entire 20 minutes and many applicants wrap up their consultation prior to this. A few deaneries use 10 minutes for this exercise, which is similar to the average GP consultation length. Deaneries vary in whether or not the examiner will give you a warning before your time runs out. Your examiner should tell you at the beginning of the consultation, if not simply ask. The examiner will remain silent for the remainder of the assessment. At this point, the role-player will be waiting outside the room and you will be asked to call them into the room.

The patient should be called into the room using the name given on the brief. Do not abbreviate it or use the first name only. Remember to introduce yourself clearly.

Some applicants fumble their first few words, so it is important that you practise an opening line that you are comfortable with. For example:

- 'I'm Dr Jones, a junior doctor here. How can I help you?'

- 'My name's Dr Jones, I'm a junior doctor here. What can I do for you today?'

Never underestimate the importance of first impressions. Your first steps towards building a rapport with the role-player start from when you welcome them into your room and have them seated. You should sound warm, inviting and sincere in your greeting and opening statement. You should appear comfortable and natural in your approach. That can be easier said than done with an examiner in the room, but try your best to focus.

Once you have said your opening statement, allow the role-player time to speak. Do not interrupt. Listen, observe and use encouraging body language. The opening statement, often referred to as the patient's monologue, will give you lots of clues. For example, their reason for presenting, their mood, their manner, their expectations and much more. It may feel like they are talking for an eternity during the assessment, but on average most patients 'run out of puff' within 30 seconds if left uninterrupted. Patients often report that they feel hurried or that the doctor is not listening if they are interrupted, which results in reduced patient co-operation and satisfaction. So be aware of this and do not rush them.

The role player acting as the patient will also have read a brief about the consultation. They have guidance on how to behave, appear, what to say or not, and how to respond. They are highly skilled and can display a variety of emotions. You should listen attentively to everything they say. There may be clues or hidden agendas, which you will have to pick up on and probe further into. The role player may not offer certain information unless you ask a specific or probing question and they feel a good enough rapport to open up to you.

You will have to manage the time efficiently and bring the consultation to a close. So do not be caught out by having to end the consultation abruptly.

Areas to cover in the CONSULTation

There are many consultations models and your style of consultation will be something which you develop over time. There are several models which identify stages of working through a consultation. But during the stress of an exam situation, it can be difficult to remember some of these.

We have devised a mnemonic to help you remember the fundamental points: 'CONSULT'. It serves as a simple guide of areas to include, particularly in case you become flustered and need something on which to anchor your thoughts.

The 'CONSULT' model for the simulation exercise

C	Create suitable and safe environment
O	Opening statements
N	Navigate the history - include ideas, concerns and expectations
S	Significant conditions/summarize
U	Understanding – check role-player understands
L	Liaise with role-player to achieve shared management plan
T	Tie up the consultation in a time and safety net

You should use this mnemonic to work through your consultations. The worked examples which follow are structured using this mnemonic so you can see it in action.

How to do well

The simulation exercise causes anxiety among many applicants. It has numerous variables and potential for pitfalls. Again, you must practise, practise, practise and then practise some more in order to feel prepared for whatever the exercise may throw at you on the day. You should prepare for this exercise with colleagues and obtain feedback about your performance and interaction with the group. Use the example marking scheme to help you assess one another and develop your skills.

It is worthwhile to have a few phrases in your mind to help you sound slick. For example, opening statements, how to summarize or progress the discussion and how to close the discussion. It is also helpful to practise a few phrases to help with difficult situations you might come across on the day or in case you become nervous. For example, how to manage an angry role-player or a depressed, quiet individual. Be prepared to be flexible and adapt to any situation. You will need to think on your feet and respond appropriately and professionally throughout this exercise.

Remember – actions speak louder than words. So don't forget your body language and physically interaction with the group. The examiner will be assessing this and will have view of your facial expressions too.

Your non-verbal communication skills and interaction with the group will be assessed throughout this exercise. Polish up on these skills to enhance the group dynamic and score you extra marks. To help with your non-verbal communication, remember the following helpful pointers:

- Be calm, composed and confident.
- Sit up and lean forward at the table, as if you are about to eat a meal.
- Avoid slouching or leaning back, particularly while a colleague is talking, because this can demonstrate disinterest.
- Demonstrate active listening skills and show that you are concentrating when your colleagues are speaking.
- Maintain good eye contact with whoever is speaking.
- Give encouraging nods and smiles.
- Use your hands to help you communicate and appear more natural. For example, if trying to establish consensus on a particular point you could use a thumbs up to help appear inviting and relaxed. But, beware not to flap your hands around too much while speaking because this could demonstrate nervousness.

Summary of how to do well

- If required, rearrange the furniture. At the very least, make a point of noting and commenting on the layout if no changes are required or possible.
- Build a good rapport, be warm and friendly.
- Invite and encourage the role-player to talk, while you listen attentively and display active listening skills.
- Avoid using jargon or complex medical terminology.
- Check the role-player's understanding and always invite the them to ask questions.
- Be honest if you do not know the answer to a question. Offer to find out the answer and that you will inform the patient later.
- Always offer patient information leaflets, websites or groups from which the role-player could obtain more information.
- Safety net and offer follow up if appropriate.

Common themes

Your consultation could relate to anything encountered in clinical practice! The scenario could be in a general practice or hospital setting, such as an outpatient clinic. However, some common themes for scenarios are listed below:

- explaining a diagnosis or procedure
- explaining a treatment or management plan
- breaking bad news
- handling an angry, bereaved or demanding patient or colleague
- handling a complaint
- handling a mistake or error
- handling impact of a disease
- managing psychosocial issues
- managing occupational issues.

On reading the brief, it may initially seem like a straightforward case, but there is likely to be more to unravel. You will have to explore the role-player's ideas and concerns in order to find out more and discover their underlying agenda. Asking open and sensitive probing questions should help you reveal and address the deeper issues, which will help you score higher.

You must remember that irrespective of the theme for your consultation, the GP NPS criteria against which you are being assessed remain the same. So do not be put off when you read the brief. For example, do not be flustered if you cannot remember exactly how to manage a particular clinical diagnosis. You must aim to demonstrate your skills in relation to the GP NPS.

Worked examples

The worked examples which follow will give you ideas about how to approach the consultations and give you insight into skills to demonstrate and how.

Worked example 1

Information for applicant

You are an SHO in a gynaecology outpatient clinic in a hospital setting.

> *Mrs Jefferies is a 60-year-old smoker, who was referred by her GP 5 weeks ago with post-menopausal bleeding. She was seen in clinic and booked for an ultrasound which showed a very thickened endometrium. She was subsequently booked for endometrial sampling and hysteroscopy 2 weeks ago. You expect to see her today with the results and histology following her investigations. However, she has not had the investigations nor received a date yet. She is angry with the delay and concerned she has cancer.*

Write your pre-consultation thoughts and notes below:

Information for role player (*not* to be read by the applicant)

You are Mrs Jefferies, a 60-year-old cleaner.

You experienced the menopause aged 50 years, but noticed bleeding from your vagina 5 weeks ago and went to see your GP immediately. You were referred by your GP and promptly had an ultrasound scan and were seen in a gynaecology clinic. You were told that the lining of your uterus is thickened which needs to be swiftly investigated for endometrial cancer. You do not fully understand the tests to be done, but you have been waiting weeks to hear from the hospital with an appointment.

You are extremely anxious. You work as a cleaner in a hospice where you have heard about some patients' diagnoses being missed in the first instance. You have read that endometrial cancer can be operated on by hysterectomy if picked up early. You are worried that you have cancer and it could be spreading. You are normally well and not had to call upon the NHS before, but you feel very let down and disappointed by the system. You fear that you may be diagnosed with endometrial cancer too late and it could be inoperable.

You do not have any children. Your social support network consists of your sister and your neighbour. You had another sister who died 3 years ago from breast cancer spreading to her bones. You fear that you may be diagnosed with endometrial cancer too late and it could be inoperable.

This scenario deals with a delayed investigation and potentially a delayed diagnosis of cancer. It involves managing a challenging consultation and assesses your ability to address the issues and patient's fears.

Key points for example 1

C *Create functional/safe environment*

Check you are happy with the table and chair configuration. You may wish to comment that in some hospital settings the patient is seated opposite a table, rather than at the corner of a table in general practice.

O *Opening statements*

Welcome Mrs Jefferies into the room and introduce yourself as per the brief.

Allow Mrs Jefferies to voice her anger and disappointment with the system.

Apologise early for the delay. For example, 'I'm sorry about the unexpected delay. I agree it's frustrating that the investigation has not yet happened and I'm very sorry.'

Demonstrate that you understand her anger and acknowledge her concerns. Explain that you are also disappointed that the investigation date has not been arranged and acknowledge that it is essential for a diagnosis. Doing this early within the consultation will help you develop a rapport with the patient.

Apologise again for the delay and your non-verbal communication should demonstrate that you are genuinely concerned and sorry.

N *Navigate the history*

Check the patient's contact details, particularly address. This may have changed and the appointment sent to the wrong address.

Explore her expectations now that a delay has occurred. Sometimes patients want the problem to just be rectified urgently, while others also wish to make a complaint. For example, 'I'll address the delay as a matter of urgency to make sure your investigations are done. Do you have any other concerns or expectations?'

Explore Mrs Jefferies fears. Discuss with Mrs Jefferies her fears about a delayed diagnosis. She may also bring up lack of knowledge of the investigations.

Explore her social support. Acknowledge that she appears very anxious and suggest that she brings someone with her for support at her next appointment.

S *Significant issues/summarize*

Ultimately, a potential diagnosis of cancer has yet to be made and you need to have the investigations done. You should aim to book Mrs Jefferies on to the next list for investigation. You could offer to do this while she remains in the clinic, or offer to call the patient later today with the date, time, etc.

You should also enquire about her current symptoms, particularly in case they have worsened. Is she bleeding more, is she anaemic, does she require admission?

U *Understanding – check role-player's understanding*

Check Mrs Jefferies understanding of the investigations. Check she understands what will be done next.

L *Liaise with role-player to achieve shared management plan*

Formulate an action plan which is mutually acceptable.

Mrs Jefferies may wish to make a formal complaint, in which case you will need to inform her of the local complaints procedure and/or the patient advice and liaison service (PALS).

T *Tie up the consultation in a time and safety net*

Conclude the consultation by apologising again and then reassure her that the investigations will be done and followed up swiftly.

Safety net by advising her to seek medical attention if her symptoms worsen or if she has any concerns.

Worked example 2

Information for Applicant

You are an SHO in a busy Accident and Emergency department.

Katy Colson is a 20-year-old law student. She was brought to hospital following a paracetamol overdose. She had self-confessed the overdose to her flatmate after she was found vomiting. She had taken 10 paracetamol tablets and no other substances. Her paracetamol levels are below the treatment line. Her blood tests are all normal and she does not show any signs suggestive of liver damage. She reports not wanting to kill herself. But the nurse looking after her is concerned and wants you to assess her.

Write your pre-consultation thoughts and notes below:

Information for role player *(not to be read by the applicant)*

You are Katy Colson, a 20-year-old law student.

You have been finding it increasingly difficult to cope with the work and revision pressure at university. You recently failed your end of year exams. You feel that you always try your hardest, but it is never enough.

Your mother passed away 2 months ago from a sudden heart attack aged only 45 years. She was a heavy smoker of 50 cigarettes a day. Her wish was to see you graduate as a lawyer.

You live with your flatmate, who you trust and get on well with. You broke up with your boyfriend last month because you wanted to concentrate more on your work.

You have been unable to concentrate or sleep properly for the past 2 months. You feel low in mood and have a very poor appetite. You feel useless having failed this recent exam. You are normally fit and well with no past psychiatric history. You have no delusions or hallucinations. You do not smoke or drink alcohol.

You feel that life is too difficult and not worth living, but you had not planned to take the overdose. You had no intention to commit suicide. You are not sure why you took an overdose, but think it was a cry for help. You recognize that you need support and help to get through your difficulties.

Note – you should avoid eye contact and seem distant with your body language. You may cry if you feel comfortable to open up to the applicant.

This scenario assesses your ability to manage psychosocial issues. You will be required to display a high level of communication skills and respond appropriately to the patient's problems.

Key points for example 2

C   *Create functional/safe environment*

Arrange the chairs in a correct layout and avoid any barriers between you and the patient. Beware of your own safety when seeing psychiatry cases. For example, the patient should not be between you and the door, so that you are able to reach the door without any obstacles should the need arise.

O   *Opening statements*

Welcome Katy Colson into the room and introduce yourself as per the brief.

It is unlikely that the patient will give you a monologue in this consultation and so you may have to initiate conversation. Have an empathetic and understanding manner. Use silences and allow Katy to talk, and use the silences to assess her body language. Adapt your position and tone to mirror hers.

Start off by asking a very open question, such as 'How are you feeling?' From this Katy may respond with either her physical feeling (i.e. nausea, abdominal pain) or her mental feeling (i.e. sad, useless) depending on which is bothering her most. However, she may blankly respond 'fine' in which case you should acknowledge that she does not seem it.

Reassure her that you are here to help.

N   *Navigate the history*

Ask if she has any physical symptoms such as nausea or abdominal pain. Clarify the history and ask about how many tablets she took and did she take any other substances or alcohol.

Explore the circumstances surrounding the overdose. Explore why and what led Katy to take the overdose. For example, had she planned the self-harm, did she know her flatmate would find her, did she induce the vomit, did she write a note? Had she intended to kill herself? Does she want to die? How does she feel about it all now? Rather than jump in and start firing off these questions, you should introduce them first by using a phase such as, 'May I ask a few questions about the overdose itself and how you feel about it?' or 'I need to ask some questions about the overdose and your intentions. Is that okay?'

Demonstrate to Katy that you understand she is going through a difficult time and discuss each with her: bereavement following loss of mother, studying pressures, relationship. To start of this discussion you could say, 'You've clearly been through a lot and the past couple of months have been really hard, anyone in your shoes would naturally be upset. How do you feel about …?'

Explore her social and support network. For example, 'How are you getting on with friends/family?' or 'Which activities do you do? Are there any you particularly enjoy … Who do you do these with?' Can she talk to anybody senior or a mentor at university.

Explore Katy's expectations now. Does she feel she needs help? Explain to the patient that help is available and also suggest that she contacts her supervisor and counsellors at university.

You should have a respectful, calm and supportive manner throughout the consultation. Do not come across as being judgemental. Getting the right tone of voice is essential. Remember this is likely to be her first meaningful contact with medical services and help. If your attitude is not receptive then she may not seek any further help. Allow silences within the consultation, these are helpful. Allow Katy a chance to reflect. You should use encouraging nods and could say '… Tell me more', '… I can see how tough this is for you' or '… Take your time.'

S   *Significant issues/summarize*

All doctors should be able to conduct a psychosocial and psychiatric mental state assessment to ascertain risk.

Enquire about any past psychiatric history, suicidal ideation, hallucinations, persecutory delusions, paranoia, sleep pattern disturbance, reduced appetite, poor concentration and libido. Some of these points may get covered when you explore her symptoms earlier in the consultation. But if not, you must remember to ask specifically even if you suspect the answer to be No. You may want to 'normalize' your questions by putting them into context for her and saying that these are routine questions that we ask patients.

Explain to Katy that paracetamol overdose can cause severe liver damage and the effects are not immediately obvious. Explain that her blood tests are normal. She is unlikely to have any long-term severe side effects given the amount taken and that she vomited afterwards.

U   *Understanding – check role-player's understanding*

Check Katy understands why she should seek support and help.

L   *Liaise with role-player to achieve shared management plan*

Formulate an action plan which is mutually acceptable.

Agree with Katy that her GP will receive information about her attendance to hospital and that she should visit her GP to discuss things further.

T   *Tie up the consultation in a time and safety net*

Invite Katy to ask any questions or share anything. You could conclude the consultation with support and reassurance.

You should safety net by advising her to seek to discuss things further with her GP and supervisor at university.

Worked example 3

Information for applicant

You are an FY2 doctor in a general practice surgery.

> *Mr Jason Keane, a 32-year-old estate agent, has come to see you having been discharged from hospital 1 week previously. He is normally fit and well.*
>
> *From the discharge summary, you learn that he was admitted having experienced a solitary fit. His ECG, CT head scan and EEG were all normal and he was informed not to drive for 6 months in accordance with DVLA guidance. He would like to discuss this with you.*

Write your pre-consultation thoughts and notes below:

_____

_____

_____

_____

_____

_____

Information for role player (*not* to be read by the applicant)

You are Mr Jason Keane, a 32-year-old estate agent.

> *You were admitted to hospital following a solitary fit after a night out with friends. You were discharged from hospital 1 week ago and told on discharge that you cannot drive for 6 months. You feel well in yourself and have experienced no further fits. You do not understand why you cannot drive and fear that you will lose your job which requires you to drive to clients' properties.*
>
> *You do not normally drink to excess but it was your friend's 30th birthday and you became drunk. You think the fit was alcohol-related. You normally drink only two pints of beer per week. You do not smoke. You have no past medical history and are normally very well. You have recently got married and bought a new flat.*
>
> *Your job involves a lot of driving and you have not been back to work since you were discharged. You want to return to work. You are worried you could lose your job if you cannot drive. You have not considered a temporary change of role within the company which does not involve driving, nor have you considered discussing the situation with your employer. You are turning to your GP for advice and explanation of why you cannot drive for 6 months.*
>
> *At the end of the consultation, you are receptive of the GPs advice to consult your employers. You will display annoyance if the doctor does not give you a satisfactory explanation or assistance.*

This scenario tests your ability to manage the impact of disease and occupational issues. It also requires you to act within professional and legal boundaries.

Key points for example 3

C	*Create functional/safe environment*
	Check you are happy with the table and chair configuration. Ensure there is no barrier or table between you and the patient.
O	*Opening statements*
	Welcome Mr Keane into the room and introduce yourself as per the brief and ask how you can help. Allow him to inform you of his presentation today.
	Alternatively, you could open by acknowledging his recent admission to hospital and asking how he is.
N	*Navigate the history*
	Explore Mr Keane's understanding of why he was admitted and investigated.
	Explore how Mr Keane has been since discharge. Has he had any further fits? There is little value for you to dwell on the fit which led to his admission as this has been thoroughly investigated during his hospital stay.
	Express that you understand that being banned from driving is very difficult for him and his work. Explore his occupation. Explore his expectations about driving and his occupation. Enquire whether he understands why he cannot drive and if he has been informed of the DVLA regulations. For example, 'I see that being banned from driving is causing you difficulties with work, but do you understand why you aren't allowed to drive?'
	Explore Mr Keane's concerns about being unable to drive for 6 months. Has he informed work about his fit or ban and how these could be addressed? For example, 'Have you tried discussing with your employer that you're not allowed to drive? It would be worthwhile, because they may be able to help by temporarily altering your role so you don't need to drive or find another solution.'
S	*Significant issues/summarize*
	Remind him that his investigations were normal, however he ultimately had a fit. This means that he is legally banned from driving for 6 months. You should explain that this is the law. It is for his own and public safety. Mr Keane's view that the fit was alcohol-related is not accepted by the DVLA as an excuse. The 6-month ban also applies to alcohol-related seizures. You must also explain that it is his responsibility to inform the DVLA and he must not drive until he fulfils their guidelines. Inform Mr Keane that if he does not inform the DVLA and continues to drive, then you will have to inform the DVLA.
	Mr Keane's employment is a significant concern for him and so this must be addressed. You should advise him to discuss his situation with his employer. Advise him to negotiate with his employer an alternative role for the duration of the ban, for example remaining office-based. You could offer to contact his occupational health doctor or provide a letter which may help.
U	*Understanding – check role-player's understanding*
	Check Mr Keane understands that he must not drive. He must also inform the DVLA. Reiterate that you will have no option but to inform the DVLA yourself if he does not and continues to drive.
L	*Liaise with role-player to achieve shared management plan*
	Formulate an action plan which is mutually acceptable.
	Negotiate a shared management plan regarding Mr Keane's discussion with his employer and if he would like you to help by writing a letter in support.
T	*Tie up the consultation in a time and safety net*
	Conclude the consultation by displaying your understanding of how this is difficult for him. You should safety net by asking him to return next week or sooner if required, so that you can follow up on the advice, support him and check that he has informed the DVLA.

Worked example 4

Information for applicant

You are a junior doctor in a gastroenterology outpatient clinic.

> *Your next patient is Mr Elkins, a 68-year-old retired chef. He was referred by his GP with a change in bowel habit and weight loss. Digital rectal examination was normal. Your consultant performed a colonoscopy and biopsy on Mr Elkins last week. Histology revealed colorectal carcinoma. Your consultant has been called away to an emergency case. Mr Elkins is seeing you in clinic today for his results.*

Write your pre-consultation thoughts and notes below:

Information for role player (*not* to be read by the applicant)

You are Mr Elkins, a 68-year-old retired chef.

> *You have noticed that your bowels have not been the same since you returned from a Caribbean cruise with your wife 6 months ago. You had suffered with diarrhoea during this trip and took imodium. You then felt constipated and took some laxatives. Since then, your bowels have never really settled and you've been like a yo-yo between constipation and diarrhoea. You had been purchasing laxatives and imodium over the counter, but became fed up and went to your GP requesting them on repeat prescription so it would be free. However, your GP referred you to gastroenterology.*

> *This seemed rather excessive to you, particularly when you saw the consultant and he suggested a colonoscopy. From your consultation with the consultant last week, your understanding is that the colonoscopy was to look for any 'lumps' in the bowel which might be causing the diarrhoea and constipation. You do not correlate these 'lumps' with cancer.*

> *Your wife had read in a book that this may be cancer, but you had reassured yourself that it could not be because it all started when you were on the cruise. You have no past medical history and have always had normal regular bowels before.*

> *Your wife is accompanying you to the appointment and is anxious. You reassure her.*

> *You are taken aback and stunned by the diagnosis. Your initial reaction is of denial. There must be some mistake in the report or a mix up. You ask to speak with the consultant who saw you last week. You accept that he is not available yet due to an emergency case. But you would like to see him. As the consultation goes on, you gradually accept the diagnosis and would like to know what happens next.*

This scenario involves breaking bad news. This is an area commonly tested, and such consultations can be very challenging. You should adapt your approach in response to the patient's reaction.

Key points for example 4

C   *Create functional/safe environment*

Check you are happy with the table and chair configuration. In reality, you should ensure a quiet environment with minimal disturbance. You would ask a colleague to hold your bleep for a short while so that you are not called away during this consultation.

O   *Opening statements*

Welcome Mr Elkins into the room and introduce yourself as per the brief.

Ask if Mr Elkins has anyone/a relative accompanying him. For the stage 3 assessment, the answer will usually be No, but it is good practice to ask and invite in the relative if the patient consents.

Invite him to inform you of why he is in clinic today. This may help you gauge his insight and level of anxiety, if any. Sometimes, patients are visibly very anxious and you should acknowledge this valuable non-verbal cue. You could also ask how he has been since his last appointment.

N   *Navigate the history*

Explore Mr Elkins' understanding of why he had the colonoscopy. Ask what he was told at his last appointment and what had been discussed about the potential causes of his change in bowel habit. What is he expecting?

S   *Significant issues/summarize*

Explain the histology findings of colorectal cancer. Use a 'warning shot' before giving the definitive diagnosis. For example, 'I'm afraid I have some bad news' or 'I'm sorry, but the results show (diagnosis)'. Allow a moment for this to sink in.

Encourage the patient to voice their opinion and view. Explore the situation from the patient's perspective. For example, 'Have you heard of ... before?' or 'Understandably this is a lot to take on board, I'd like to hear your thoughts' or 'Share your concerns with me'. You should respond appropriately to the patient's comments and concern. The patient's response may be of anger or denial and you should explain that these reactions are natural. If the patient responds with anger or denial, do not become defensive or abrupt in return. Remain calm, assertive and supportive.

Answer Mr Elkins questions truthfully. He may have questions about the diagnosis, surgery or dying. Do not pretend to be an expert or give false hope. Use appropriate language to suit the patient's level of understanding and avoid jargon. Give information in small chunks and use short sentences. Avoid overloading the patient with too much information. If the patient directly asks 'How long do I have doctor?' you should be honest that you do not know. You must avoid giving any precise figure. It would be acceptable for you to acknowledge that this is an understandable concern to him, but at the moment you do not have enough information and would need to await further investigation (i.e. staging CT scan) and see how he responds to treatment. You could also offer for him to see the consultant, perhaps after the CT, who could answer his question with more clarity.

Summarize as you go along. Acknowledge that this is a lot of information to take on board and offer to go through any information again. Ask if Mr Elkins has any questions as you go along. There is no value in you talking away if the patient is not following the conversation.

Signpost to help the consultation have structure. This will help Mr Elkins follow the consultation. For example, 'We'll move on now to discuss what will happen next and then I have some leaflets for you.'

U   *Understanding – check role-player's understanding*

Check Mr Elkins' understanding of the diagnosis and situation. Offer to answer any more questions he may have.

Throughout the consultation you should take opportunities to reassure Mr Elkins that he will be supported both physically and mentally with this condition, not only by the gastroenterology team, but the multidisciplinary team, such as specialist nurses and his GP.

L   *Liaise with role-player to achieve shared management plan*

Formulate an action plan which is mutually acceptable.

Remember this is an exercise about breaking bad news and not about colorectal cancer. Your communication and negotiation skills are being tested. This patient requires a staging CT scan next, but your clinical management plan is not the 'be all and end all' of the consultation. If there is something you do not know about colorectal cancer then offer to find out and get back to him. If you do not know the answer to a particular question, be honest and say, 'I'm sorry I don't know the answer to this question but I'll discuss with my consultant and get back to you.' Mr Elkins may wish to see your consultant. If so, do not be obstructive, but do ask if there is anything more you can help with. You should explain that your consultant is busy with an emergency case. You should negotiate with Mr Elkins when he would be able to see the consultant.

Some patients take longer than others to reach the 'acceptance phase' and you should acknowledge this. For example, 'This has clearly come as a shock to you. I suggest we meet again next week so you have some time for this to sink in and we can answer any questions and discuss treatment options.'

Trying to reach a shared management plan can be difficult if the patient is still shocked or not communicative. Always try to encourage the patient to interact and be involved. For example, 'How does this plan sound to you?' or 'Does this sound reasonable?' Avoid using clichés or trying to make light-hearted irrelevant discussion, such as 'Are you happy with this plan?' or 'Lovely sunshine for you to enjoy.'

Always offer support and inform the patient of specialist nurses or recognized help groups for the particular condition.

T   *Tie up the consultation in a time and safety net*

Give Mr Elkins a patient information leaflet towards the end of the consultation. Ask him to read it and jot down any questions he may have so you can answer them in the next consultation. Follow up for this patient will be important to help him come to terms with the diagnosis.

Worked example 5

Information for applicant

You are a junior doctor in a general practice surgery.

> *Three weeks ago you saw 14-year-old Chantelle Bennett who wanted to start the oral contraceptive pill. She was in a relationship with a boy in her class at school who she has known for 3 years. She is competent and meets Fraser criteria. She could not be persuaded to inform her parents. She has no past medical history. You discussed her contraceptive options and advise regarding safe sex and condom use. She was started on the oral contraceptive pill (OCP).*

> *Chantelle's mother, Mrs Bennett, is angry and has come to see you today because you started Chantelle on the OCP.*

Write your pre-consultation thoughts and notes below:

Information for role player (*not* to be read by the applicant)

You are Mrs Bennett, mother of Chantelle Bennett.

> *You have been concerned for months that your daughter is in a sexual relationship with a boy in her class. You have been worried that she will fall pregnant at a young age and ruin her life. You have tried discussing this with Chantelle, but she is very obstructive.*

> *You recently found an empty packet of the OCP in Chantelle's bedroom. You confronted Chantelle, but she refused to tell you anything. You are worried that she is too young for all of this and that she may contract some infection, like HIV.*

> *You feel angry yet helpless and powerless. You turn to the GP for more information about why Chantelle was started on contraception so young and without the mother knowing.*

This scenario deals with confidentiality and consent. It also touches on child protection which is vitally important. If there are any concerns about Chantelle's safety, then local policy should be followed for disclosure and discussion with the child protection lead.

Key points for example 5

C *Create functional/safe environment*

Check the table and chair configuration, and move any barriers between you and the patient. In reality, you would be mindful not to have Chantelle's notes open on the computer screen because the mother could potentially see them.

O *Opening statements*

Welcome Mrs Bennett into the room and introduce yourself as per the brief.

Invite Mrs Bennett to say why she is here to see you. For example, 'How can I help you today?'

Listen attentively to Mrs Bennett's concerns.

Apologise early for the way Mrs Bennett is feeling and acknowledge her anger. Display empathy and understanding, for example 'As a caring parent this must be frustrating and difficult for you, and I understand that you must feel left in the dark.'

N *Navigate the history*

Explore what and how much Mrs Bennett already knows. Be mindful not to disclose any new information to her. Explore Mrs Bennett's specific concerns.

S *Significant issues/summarize*

Does she have any worries about child safety or abuse? Does she know the partner? Why is she concerned about HIV in particular? For example, 'Do you have any particular worries about her safety?'

Tactfully explain to Mrs Bennett that you have a duty to confidentiality to Chantelle and cannot discuss the case without Chantelle's consent. For example, 'I appreciate your concerns, but I have a duty to maintain confidentiality to all my patients, including Chantelle and yourself. I'm sorry I can't discuss any details with you without her consent.' Acknowledge that you can see and admire her sense of parental responsibility. Explain to Mrs Bennett the importance of building a trusting doctor–patient relationship with Chantelle.

Remember that child protection is of highest priority. If you or the mother suspects any form of child abuse or child safety concern, then this must be acted upon immediately in the child's best interest.

Suggest and encourage the mother to attend with Chantelle. Explain that you would be willing to discuss the case with Chantelle's consent and her present.

Explain to Mrs Bennett that your actions were in Chantelle's best interest and medicolegally Chantelle is able to make such decisions, without parental knowledge or consent. Reassure her that Chantelle was appropriately advised and counselled. Reassure Mrs Bennett that you discussed condom use and protection against sexually transmitted infections, as you do with all your contraception consultations.

U *Understanding – check role-player's understanding*

Check that Mrs Bennett understands that you treated Chantelle in her best interests and child safety issues are always considered. Also check that Mrs Bennett understands your duty of confidentiality to Chantelle, so that she does not leave feeling that you are being obstructive or hiding something. For example, 'I hope you understand that we're acting in Chantelle's best interests and as doctors, we have a duty to our patients and don't want her to come to any harm either.'

L *Liaise with role-player to achieve shared management plan*

Formulate an action plan which is mutually acceptable.

Reiterate that you would be happy to see Mrs Bennett and Chantelle together during a consultation. Highlight to Mrs Bennett that you will continue to encourage Chantelle to inform her mother of decisions to help obtain support and build a good relationship.

T *Tie up the consultation in a time and safety net*

Offer Mrs Bennett the opportunity to ask any other questions or raise other concerns. If she is satisfied, close the consultation by thanking her for coming to see you today and that you hope to see her with Chantelle in the future.

Worked example 6

Information for applicant

You are an FY2 doctor in a general practice surgery.

> *Mr Kevin Lohan is a 48-year-old factory worker. He comes to see you in the hypertension clinic. He attends today having missed two previous appointments for the clinic. He has essential hypertension diagnosed 18 months ago.*

You note from his records that his blood pressure has been gradually increasing over the past 12 months. He is on a low dose of ramipril, but you notice that he has not been ordering his repeat prescription regularly. You doubt his adherence and hope to raise this issue in today's consultation.

Write your pre-consultation thoughts and notes below:

_____

_____

_____

_____

Information for role player (*not* to be read by the applicant)

You are Mr Kevin Lohan, a 48-year-old factory worker.

> *You were diagnosed with hypertension 18 months ago. You don't really believe the diagnosis because you always feel so well, but the GP started you on some tablets (ramipril). You took these tablets for the first 4–6 months, but felt no different so you stopped taking them and now only rarely use them.*
>
> *You hate visiting the GP surgery because you're not an 'ill' kind of person. You have no symptoms of high blood pressure and feel healthy.*
>
> *Only disclose to the doctor that you rarely take your medication if he/she makes you feel comfortable enough to do so. The doctor will explain to you why you must be on the tablets and take them. You do not want to take them. You do not have any side effects or concern about them, but you simply do not believe the diagnosis. You do not see why you should take medications for a problem you don't have or for which you have no symptoms.*
>
> *You will negotiate and agree to trial the tablets for a couple of months with regular blood pressure monitoring. If there is an improvement in your blood pressure over this time, you would accept the diagnosis and continue treatment.*

This scenario addresses poor adherence and chronic disease management. It highlights the importance of patient education and empowerment to help improve their understanding and cooperation with management.

Key points for example 6

C   *Create functional/safe environment*

Check you are happy with the table and chair configuration.

O   *Opening statements*

Welcome Mr Kevin Lohan into the room and introduce yourself as per the brief.

Commend him for coming to the clinic today. For example, 'It's good to see you here today.' Do not start by reprimanding him and highlighting that he did not attend previous appointments – this will not get you off on the right foot.

Ask him an open question first, such as 'How's your high blood pressure?' or 'How's your blood pressure been?' This will give you valuable insight into his perception of it.

N   *Navigate the history*

Enquire about how he finds taking his tablets. Does ramipril suit him? Has he had any side effects from it? You should give Mr Lohan ample opportunity to admit himself that he is not adhering with the medication. For example, 'How are the tablets suiting you, any problems?' Pause and allow him the chance to open up. There could be several reasons why he is not taking his medications. For example, denial, side effects, perceived lack of efficacy, uses alternative therapies, fear of dependence, forgetful, unable to obtain them or unsure how to take them.

If he shares with you that he is not taking the tablets and explains why, then explore these concerns further with him. Explore his understanding and knowledge of hypertension. Address his concerns and the importance of taking the medication. Try to 'normalize' his feelings and express that his response is natural, particularly given that hypertension is not visible. However, you must highlight that this is because Mr Lohan still has early disease. Does he know about the effects and dangers of high blood pressure? You should mention the increased risk of stroke, ischaemic heart disease and heart failure. Has anyone referred to it as a 'silent killer'?

If he replies that everything is fine, then you will need to raise the subject of adherence yourself. Start off by highlighting that his blood pressure seems to be getting progressively worse. For example, 'Looking at your blood pressure readings, I'm concerned that your blood pressure is getting worse.' Pause again, giving him another chance to open up, then offer potential explanations why this may be the case with poor adherence being one of them.

S   *Significant issues/Summarize*

Exclude any potential red flags or end organ damage, such as headache or proteinuria. Indicate that you would also like to repeat his blood pressure today.

Stress to him the importance of treating high blood pressure and acknowledge that it can be difficult given that it is 'invisible'.

Summarize what you have said to Mr Lohan and ask, 'Do you have any questions at this point before we move on?'

U   *Understanding – check role-player's understanding*

This should not be done as a 'test' for the patient. But you could invite him to relay his understanding of hypertension. For example, 'I feel it's important that you understand hypertension, and that way we can help each other when managing it. What do you feel you've gained or learnt from our discussion today?'

L   *Liaise with role-player to achieve shared management plan*

Formulate an action plan which is mutually acceptable.

You should advise the patient to take the ramipril daily as prescribed. This is likely to be a big step for him, so seek out his expectations. You may need to negotiate a closely monitored trial period and then re-evaluate his blood pressure, symptoms and medication.

Ultimately, if the managed plan for Mr Lohan is not patient-centred or to his satisfaction, then he will simply not take the medication. So you should demonstrate that you are trying to help him and reach a safe agreed management plan together.

T   *Tie up the consultation in a time and safety net*

Ensure that you arrange follow up for Mr Lohan. Ideally, he should come back to see you for continuity and to help maintain the rapport. Advise him to come in prior to the arranged follow up should he have any questions or concerns about what you've discussed or his medications.

Give him a patient information leaflet to summarize your discussion about hypertension.

If you have any time remaining, you could also discuss other health promotion areas, such as smoking, weight, exercise and diet.

Worked example 7

Information for applicant

You are a junior doctor in a general practice surgery.

You are running very behind schedule today, because the senior partner has been called away on an emergency, so you are seeing his booked patients too.

Your next patient is Miss Jenny Pickle, a 19-year-old secretary. Her appointment time was almost an hour ago. Her last consultation was regarding her eczema. She was seen by the senior partner who is not here today. According to the computer entry for that consultation, he had restarted her on topical emollients, which she had not required since she was a toddler.

She comes today requesting referral for laser therapy to 'cure' her eczema. She has read about this on the internet. It is new and not available on the NHS as far as you are aware. You do not refer her.

Write your pre-consultation thoughts and notes below:

Information for role player (*not* to be read by the applicant)

You are Miss Jenny Pickle, a 19-year-old secretary.

You suffered with eczema as a baby but seemed to 'grow out of it'. You are a secretary and noticed that your hands became very dry, itchy and sore. You visited the GP recently who gave you some emollient cream, which sometimes helps sooth the soreness but generally has been of little benefit.

You recently read on the internet about laser therapy for eczema and you would like your GP to refer you for this. It was an American website, but you know it is available in the UK.

You persist for the GP to refer you, at the very least you feel you should be referred to a specialist. The GP declines to refer you. You become very upset if the explanations given are not satisfactory or not conveyed with compassion.

This scenario relates to coping under pressure, managing a patient's expectations and negotiation skills. It also touches on practising evidence-based medicine.

Key points for example 7

C   *Create functional/safe environment*

Check you are happy with the table and chair configuration. Despite running behind schedule, the environment should be clutter free and organized.

O   *Opening statements*

Welcome Miss Jenny Pickle into the room and introduce yourself as per the brief.

Thank Jenny for her patience. For example, 'Thank you for waiting.' If she expresses obvious annoyance or anger with the wait, then you should acknowledge this by following up with 'I understand that the wait can be frustrating.' This should be enough to pacify the patient and set off the consultation on the right note. It is important to note the phraseology used here. Saying 'Thank you for waiting' rather than 'I'm sorry about the wait' is considered more positive. It is regarded as a compliment to the patient and is likely to diffuse their potential anger, so the patient is likely to be friendly in return. In contrast, some people respond to 'I'm sorry about the wait' with more anger and are hostile because they feel they have a right to be.

Enquire about Jenny's presentation today, 'How can I help you?'

Listen attentively to Jenny's opening statement. She is coming to you with this new laser therapy idea and so she is likely to have read information about it. Her approach may be to sell the idea of it to you so that you will refer her.

N   *Navigate the history*

Explore Jenny's understanding, knowledge and desire of the therapy. Why does she want it? Have her symptoms worsened? What is she expecting the result to be? For example, 'What are your expectations from the laser therapy?'

Enquire about her eczema. How is her eczema at the moment? Has she considered the usual treatments for eczema, if not, why? How is the eczema affecting her life?

S   *Significant issues/summarize*

Demonstrate empathy and display understanding of her difficulty with chemicals at work and her eczema, but explain that this new laser therapy is not likely to offer her cure.

You should explain to Jenny that the internet is a resource which provides general information. There is unlikely to be enough, if any, unbiased evidence in support of it. The claims of cure are likely to be commercialized hype in the interests of advertisement. Explain that the information is unlikely to be reliable or valid. Highlight that all treatments available on the NHS are thoroughly tested in clinical trials beforehand and deemed safe by reputable organizations.

You should be honest that you do not know exact details of this laser therapy, but generally speaking it may have side effects, such as burns or scarring.

You should highlight that it is not available on the NHS and could become very costly for her.

Conveying these points to her may be difficult. Do not bombard her with all of them at once. It is a case of slowly talking her through each point and allowing realization on her part.

For example, you could begin, 'I can see your interest in this therapy and why it looks appealing, but I have some concerns about it ...' Alternatively, you could start by trying to gauge her perception of the potential risks or disadvantages involved. For example, 'I can understand why you find this therapy appealing, but have you considered what the down-side or risks are?'

Other phrases may be, 'I am worried that this therapy may do you more harm than good,' 'There are side effects to laser therapy, such as burns or scarring,' 'Unfortunately, there is no evidence to support the use of such laser therapy in the treatment of mild eczema and I'm concerned about the truth in the commercial claims they advertise,' and 'I'm sorry this therapy is not available on the NHS, which means you would have to fund it and sometimes this can be very expensive.' You will have to convey these messages with clarity to ensure that your point and reasons for not referring are understood by the patient.

If the patient persists for referral, or for a second opinion, and is not convinced by your advice, then you should offer to speak with your senior/GP partner. For example, 'I'd like to discuss this with my senior colleague and seek their view first.'

You should emphasize the basic principles of eczema management and advise her to continue using the emollients. You should also remind her that there are several treatments available on the NHS which may help her eczema. For example, 'How is the emollient cream suiting you? Have you considered different options available via the NHS, such as steroid-based creams?'

U   *Understanding – check role-player's understanding*

You should demonstrate that the patient understands your concerns and reasons for not referring. This is particularly important for this scenario, because it acts as a stepping stone towards reaching a shared management plan. For example, 'I hope you can understand my concerns and the risks involved with this new therapy' or 'I'm sorry I can't refer you at this stage until I find out more about this therapy and have spoken with my senior. Can you understand that I don't wish to put you at unnecessary risk?'

L   *Liaise with role-player to achieve shared management plan*

Formulate an action plan which is mutually acceptable.

If Jenny has demonstrated understanding of your reasoning and concerns then this should be easy. If not, you could find yourself in a sticky negotiation situation where the patient is demanding to be referred.

T   *Tie up the consultation in a time and safety net*

You should thank the patient for coming to see you and remind her to continue applying the emollient. You should arrange follow up within a few days, so that you can update the patient about the outcome of your discussion with your senior colleague.

Worked example 8

Information for applicant

You are a junior doctor in a general practice surgery.

> *You saw Mrs Tomlin 3 days ago. She is a 36-year-old publican. You had received her cervical smear report which showed she has CIN III. You broke the news to Mrs Tomlin 3 days ago and referred her for urgent colposcopy.*

> *However, today you received a telephone call from the hospital saying there had been an administrative error and Mrs Tomlin's cervical smear was actually normal. They confirmed this to you by fax and sent Mrs Tomlin's correct report.*

> *You called Mrs Tomlin today asking her to attend the surgery to see you. You told her that you want to discuss her smear results, but it's nothing to worry about. You would like to inform her of the error and that her results are normal.*

Write your pre-consultation thoughts and notes below:

_____

_____

_____

_____

_____

_____

_____

_____

_____

_____

Information for role player (*not* to be read by the applicant)

You are Mrs Tomlin, a 36-year-old publican.

> *Three days ago, you were informed by the doctor that your cervical smear showed carcinoma-in-situ (CIN) III and you were referred for urgent colopscopy.*

> *You have been fraught with worry since and have been crying yourself to sleep at night. The doctor has made an appointment for you to see him/her today at the surgery. The doctor wants to discuss your result with you again. You are concerned that the doctor has more bad news for you. The doctor had said it was nothing to worry about, but you are expecting the worst.*

This scenario deals with your ability to handle an error. Depending on the patient's response, this can be a challenging consultation. You should apologise and remain professional throughout.

Key points for example 8

C *Create functional/safe environment*

Organize the chair layout so there are no barriers between you and the patient.

O *Opening statements*

Welcome Mrs Tomlin into the room and introduce yourself as per the brief.

Thank her for coming to see you at short notice.

Be open and honest from the start. Do not beat about the bush, because the patient will be anxious to know why you called her to come in. For example, 'I've received some good news from the hospital that your cervical smear result was in fact normal. I'm terribly sorry but they had unfortunately made an error with the results we discussed a few days ago.'

N *Navigate the history*

Explore and gauge Mrs Tomlin's response. She is likely to be shocked and angry yet relieved, and will have questions about the error. 'I'm very sorry that this happened, it must have been a difficult few days for you?' or 'It's a relief that your smear result was normal, but I'm sorry you had to go through this, how do you feel?'

Be understanding if the patent responds with anger. For example, 'I can see you are very angry about the error and the torment this has caused you, it is perfectly understandable.'

S *Significant issues/summarize*

Express your concerns about the error and that you will have it investigated so that similar errors can be avoided in future. For example, 'It is certainly no excuse, but sometimes mistakes can happen. I'm going to report this error so that it's formally investigated to avoid it happening again' or 'It's unfortunate that you had to go through this, but I'm going to report the error so that such errors do not occur in the future.'

Mrs Tomlin may not be satisfied by this and she may wish to lodge a complaint against the hospital. If so, you should inform her of the procedure and direct her towards PALS.

Reassure and highlight the good news to the patient. She may not be reassured and may want a repeat smear test or second opinion. This would be perfectly reasonable and you should agree to arrange this if requested.

U *Understanding – check patient's understanding*

Check that Mrs Tomlin understands that her result is normal, despite the initial error. For example, 'I hope you understand that your cervical smear result was normal and we can be positive about this.'

L *Liaise with role-player to achieve shared management plan*

Formulate an action plan which is mutually acceptable.

Highlight to Mrs Tomlin that you will ensure this error is looked into by the hospital.

You should recognize that Mrs Tomlin may not wish to have future cervical smears at this hospital, in which case you would be happy to refer her to another hospital. For example, 'For future smear tests, I'd fully understand if you would like me to refer you to a different hospital.'

Directly ask Mrs Tomlin if there is anything else she would like done or you can help with.

T *Tie up the consultation in a time and safety net*

Offer Mrs Tomlin the open opportunity to return if she would like to discuss matters further.

Worked example 9

Information for applicant

You are an FY2 doctor in a cardiology outpatient clinic in hospital.

Your next patient is Mr Frampton, a 52-year-old single businessman.

He was admitted following an acute myocardial infarction (MI) and was treated with coronary angioplasty. He was started on clopidogrel, aspirin, simvastatin, ramipril and atenolol and was discharged last week. He had no past medical history and had never been on any medication.

Mr Frampton has requested to see you today because he has some questions.

Write your pre-consultation thoughts and notes below:

Information for role player (*not* to be read by the applicant)

You are Mr Frampton, a 52-year-old single businessman.

You were discharged from hospital last week after being admitted with a myocardial infarction which was treated with coronary angioplasty. You were started on a concoction of medications, but not told how long to take these for.

Previously you have been fit and well, with no medications or admissions to hospital.

You have a stressful, hectic and unhealthy lifestyle. You smoke 15 cigarettes per day and drink at least a bottle of wine a day while with colleagues. Most weeks your diet consists of ready-meals and one or two restaurant dinners with business associates. Your weight is normal and so you have never considered the need to exercise.

You have some specific concerns which you would like the doctor to address:

- *Are all the tablets necessary now that the heart attack has been treated?*
- *How long do you have to take these medications for?*
- *Should you start some form of exercise or change your lifestyle?*
- *Is it safe for you to have sex?*
- *Is it safe for you to drive?*

This scenario deals with counselling patients regarding their treatment and health promotion. You should ensure that you use an appropriate level of language which is jargon-free and check the patient's understanding.

Key points for example 9

C   *Create functional/safe environment*

Check you are happy with the table and chair configuration. Ensure there is no barrier or table between you and the patient.

O   *Opening statements*

Welcome Mr Frampton into the room and introduce yourself as per the brief and ask how you can help.

Alternatively, you could open by acknowledging his recent admission to hospital and asking how he is now. Allow him to inform you of his presentation today.

N   *Navigate the history*

Explore Mr Frampton's understanding of his admission and the procedure. Explain using non-technique language what a myocardial infarction is.

Explain that he was started on medications to help prevent another MI in the future. Express that he must continue them for life – with the exception of clopidogrel. Go through each in turn explaining how they work and highlighting why each is important to be continued.

S   *Significant issues/summarize*

Mr Frampton has clearly come in with a shopping list of questions. All his questions are important and you should answer them with clarity.

It is important in this scenario to succinctly summarize the areas you have discussed. For example, 'I hope I've answered all your questions. The key things to remember are: (1) Continue the clopidogrel for 1 year then stop; (2) Continue taking all the other medications lifelong; (3) Don't drive for 4 weeks after your heart attack. Do you have any other questions I can help you with?'

U   *Understanding – check role-player's understanding*

Check Mr Frampton understands the areas discussed, in particular the significant issues, such as his medications and driving. For example, 'I'm glad you raised these questions, do you now understand the importance of taking your tablets every day and that you cannot drive for 4 weeks?'

L   *Liaise with role-player to achieve shared management plan*

Formulate an action plan which is mutually acceptable.

Inform Mr Frampton that his GP will have received a discharge summary about his admission to hospital and that you will also write to his GP about today's consultation and the advice you have given. Offer for the patient to return if needed, alternatively his care would be better followed up by his GP and allow continuity.

Agree with Mr Frampton that he will inform the DVLA of his MI and not drive for 4 weeks from the event.

Offer to refer Mr Frampton to the dietician for further advice regarding his diet. Also offer to refer him for smoking cessation support.

As you go along, ask Mr Frampton, 'How does this sound to you?' or 'If it's okay with you, I'd like to refer you to the dietician, etc.'

T   *Tie up the consultation in a time and safety net*

Close the consultation by offering Mr Frampton a patient information leaflet or website from where he can access more information about cardiac rehabilitation.

Worked example 10

Information for applicant

You are an SHO in a palliative care clinic.

Mr Edward Hind is a competent 74-year-old gentleman with known metastatic prostate cancer. He is fully aware of his terminal illness. He has been referred with uncontrollable bone pain. He is already on regular paracetamol, diclofenac and was recently started on morphine sulphate tablets (MST). His dose of MST has been gradually increased by his GP, however his pain has not settled. The Macmillan nurse shares with you that she often sees him sobbing in pain, but says he refuses to take his analgesia.

You see Mr Hind and explore his reasons behind refusing treatment.

Write your pre-consultation thoughts and notes below:

_____

_____

_____

_____

_____

_____

_____

Information for role player *(not to be read by the applicant)*

You are Mr Edward Hind, a 74-year-old gentleman with metastatic prostate cancer.

> *You are fully aware of your terminal illness. You have been in excruciating pain because the cancer has spread to your bones. The doctors have been trying to treat this pain with more and more morphine, but you refuse to take any morphine.*
>
> *You are scared that the morphine will make you drowsy and that you will die in your sleep. The pain is currently keeping you awake at night and you are becoming more exhausted and frail.*
>
> *You are also concerned about morphine being a sign of death. Your last surviving friend was started on morphine in a pump before he died. You have no other family or friends and he was taken away from you by the morphine. You are inwardly very afraid of dying, and you fear that the morphine will hasten this.*

This scenario addresses end-of-life issues and the fears and concerns of terminally ill patients. It also touches on consent and refusal of treatment and the importance of dealing with patient's preconceived ideas.

Key points for example 10

C   *Create functional/safe environment*

Check you are happy with the table and chair configuration.

O   *Opening statements*

Welcome Mr Hind into the room and introduce yourself as per the brief.

Ask him how he feels and how he is coping with the pain? Explain that he has been referred because people are worried about his pain? For example, 'I'm seeing you today to help with your pain, how is it?'

N   *Navigate the history*

Explore Mr Hind's pain in more detail and ask what analgesia he takes.

Explore his concerns and fears, such as 'Often patients find they have side effects or concerns about particular drugs, do you have any?'

Ask directly about the morphine, 'Do you have any particular concerns with the morphine?'

Listen to his answers and respond with understanding and compassion.

Explore his fears and try to establish where they stem from. For example, 'What makes you afraid of taking morphine?' or 'Have you had any experience of morphine previously?' You must highlight the different circumstances between the morphine pump which his friend was started on prior to passing away and the oral morphine which Mr Hind was prescribed.

When discussing his fears about death, you could ask if he would like to meet with a priest to help him address such issues. This would demonstrate you are not dismissing his concerns.

S   *Significant issues/summarize*

From your discussion, assess Mr Hind's capacity to consent or refuse treatment. If he is competent, then he has the right to refuse treatment and you must respect his wishes.

Nevertheless, you can still discuss with him the advantages and potential disadvantages of oral morphine. Mr Hind may not agree to take the morphine straight away, but he may accept support from you and the MDT.

Mr Hind's decision to refuse morphine should be respected, but you should explore other alternatives. Explore his opinions regarding other analgesics. For example, 'Have you considered any other pain relief medications?' or 'We would like to help reduce your pain, there are other alternatives to morphine which I'd like to discuss with you …'

U   *Understanding – check role-player's understanding*

Make sure Mr Hind understands that he is not alone and that he can change his mind or ask for help.

Try to dispel any myths and check Mr Hind's understanding of this.

L   *Liaise with role-player to achieve shared management plan*

A patient's refusal of certain treatment can pose a difficult dilemma. You should respect Mr Hind's refusal of morphine, and aim to reach an agreed management plan using alternative therapies.

T   *Tie up the consultation in a time and safety net*

You should ensure that Mr Hind is regularly followed up in the community by his GP and specialist nurses. The information should be communicated with the MDT to ensure everyone involved in his care can support his need.

Offer Mr Hind the opportunity to have morphine if he wishes. For example, 'Please think about our discussion today, and if at any point you would like to start on a small amount of morphine then don't hesitate – we are here to take care of you.'

Worked example 11

Information for the Applicant

You are an FY2 doctor on a busy acute medical rotation. You and another FY2 doctor meet to discuss some issues that need addressing. You both have a different issue to discuss.

The issue you want to discuss are the rota and lack of education/training as detailed below.

You feel that the acute medical shifts are unfairly divided on the rota. You have noticed that the rota co-ordinator puts the same doctor on the same shifts. This means that same doctors are always doing the early morning shift, while others always do the late evening shift. You feel this is unfair and each doctor should do a variety of shifts.

You also feel that the educational and training needs of you and your colleagues are not met. You are often unable to attend the mandatory teaching sessions. You are concerned of the impact this will have on your foundation training. You feel this rotation is for service provision only and none of your educational needs are considered.

Write your pre-meeting thoughts and notes below:

Information for the role player (*not* to be read by the applicant)

You are an FY2 doctor on a busy acute medical rotation. You are meeting with your colleague to discuss some issues you noticed. You would like to discuss the lack of senior support and annual leave provision.

You feel that there is a lack of senior support available in the department. You have often felt out of your depth and unsupported. Thankfully, there have been no errors or incidents, but the lack of senior cover is of concern to you.

You also feel that it is very difficult to organise annual leave on this rotation. Often swaps are impossible due to the rota. There is no system in place where the Trust will reimburse for annual leave days not taken at the end of the rotation. There is no system for communicating who is on annual leave and you are concerned that one day there may inadvertently be a lack of cover.

This simulation exercise addresses several important issues relating to junior doctors. More importantly, it addresses your ability to discuss and liaise with a colleague in a professional and productive manner.

Key points for example 11

- **Opening statements:** You could start off the exercise with, "Thanks for meeting. I understand we've got a few different issues we'd like to discuss, would you like to share your concerns first?" You may prioritise to discuss the 'senior support' and 'annual leave' concerns first, because they could pose potential risk to patient safety.

- **Rota:** is there any particular reason it is setup in this way? Consider its implications on learning. For example, is the doctor in the morning only being exposed to ward rounds and none of the jobs, therefore not learning how to prioritise tasks? Have other methods been tried in the past? Would a 'rolling' rota be more suitable so that each doctor is exposed to a different type of shift? Consider drawing up a potential rota which is considered suitable and discussing it with the rota-coordinator and consultants in charge.

- **Education/training:** what reasons prevent the doctors from attending the teaching? Consider if it is work-overload or lack of doctors available to cover. Are the seniors aware that it's mandatory and the impact of non-attendance on you foundation training? Consider discussing with the education centre what they could do to help.

- **Senior support:** consider the potential impact on patient safety. Consider why senior support has been lacking. For example, are there un-filled senior vacancies, are they busy with other emergency cases? Consider when senior support is most needed, is it particular times of day or for unexpected difficult cases. Has anyone completed any incident forms about the lack of senior support? You don't have to wait for a clinical error or mishap to occur before completing an incident form. Consider discussing it with the lead consultant for the department.

- **Annual leave:** often a tricky issue, but particularly concerning is the high risk of potentially lacking/no cover due to poor communication. There should be a robust system in place to identify who is on-shift at any given time. Discuss what system(s) could be introduced to rectify this. It could be a really simple solution such as one big calendar onto which each doctor marks the annual leave they have been granted, or perhaps a spreadsheet. Consider the impact this issue is having on the doctors. Is it affecting morale? Are the doctors more tired, and so at risk of making mistakes? Consider if the issue should be discussed with external organisations, such as the BMA.

- Summarize the discussion you have had and appropriately allocate tasks between you. You should agree to meet again soon and feedback on any progress.

Worked example 12

Information for the applicant

You are a GP partner and your PCT is encouraging the promotion of men's health. The PCT has offered a financial incentive to set up a men's health clinic. You and another GP partner are meeting to discuss this.

Discuss the issues and conclude with an action plan of what to do next.

Write your pre-meeting thoughts and notes below:

Information for the role player (*not* to be read by the applicant)

You are a GP partner and your PCT is encouraging the promotion of men's health. The PCT has offered a financial incentive to set up a men's health clinic. You and another GP partner are meeting to discuss this.

Discuss the issues and conclude with an action plan of what to do next.

Note – the applicant and role player briefs for this scenario are the same.

You should aim to encourage debate and discuss during the meeting. Ask appropriate questions which allow the applicant to come up with solutions or ideas. Highlight pitfalls that may arise if appropriate.

Setting up a new service allows for much debate and decision making. Therefore, it is a good topic for discussion. The points to consider when having such a discussion are given below.

Key points for example 12

- Is there a need or demand for such a service? What evidence supports this?

- Consider the advantages and disadvantages of the service.

- Who would be the stakeholders in such a service (e.g. doctors, PCT, patient forum, nurses, allied health professionals, reception staff) and what are their views?

- Identify the target population, for example age group, and aim to establish the target population size so that your aims are realistic and proportional.

- Do you have the resources available to set this up and maintain it? What would be the cost/benefit analysis?

- The consideration of resources should include: staffing, premises, funding, equipment and time.

- Ultimately a business plan for proposing a new service will need to be formulated.

- Discuss the key focus points of the service. For example, would the men's health clinic be a service for men to have a regular appointment and visit the GP, or would it focus on issues such mental health, STI prevention, healthy lifestyle promotion?

- Consider the logistics of the services. For example: when is the best time to have a men's health clinic; do you have staff available for this; what would happen if certain staff are on leave/away; how will the service be advertised and promoted, who will monitor and be responsible for the service?

- How will quality assurance be assessed? How will the success (or not) of the service be measured? You should identify the need for regular audit.

- Your meeting should give rise to lots of action points. These should be appropriately delegated between you. A follow-up meeting should be agreed (i.e. in approximately a week) to allow further discussion and a potential decision.

Worked example 13

Information for the applicant

You are an SHO in hospital. You are meeting with another SHO to discuss your concerns regarding 4 of your colleagues. Your consultant would like a summary of the discussion and your agreed action plan. You both have 2 colleagues each to discuss.

You are concerned about Dr Colin Day (Case 1). He is an ST1 doctor who recently went away for a long weekend in Greece with his friends. However, his leave had not been granted. Instead he called in sick and went on holiday. You were appalled when you found out and feel that you can no longer trust him.

You are also concerned about Dr Jasmine Randan (Case 2). She is a conscientious FY2 doctor who does not hand over jobs at the end of a shift. She feels ashamed to hand over jobs and tasks she hasn't completed. So she hands over the bleep and informs you of any unwell patients, but remains in the hospital finishing the jobs. Often she is in the hospital until very late into the evening. You do not have any concerns about her clinical work or patient safety. Your main concern is for Jasmine's wellbeing and you feel the pressure of the job may be too much for her.

Write your pre-meeting thoughts and notes below:

_____

_____

_____

_____

_____

_____

_____

_____

_____

_____

Information for the role player (*not* to be read by the applicant)

You are an SHO in hospital. You are meeting with another SHO to discuss your concerns regarding 4 of your colleagues. Your consultant would like a summary of the discussion and your agreed action plan. You both have 2 colleagues each to discuss.

You are concerned about Dr Timothy Kays (Case 3). He is an FY2 doctor who recently went through a difficult divorce. On two occasions at work, you smelt alcohol on his breath and he has appeared dishevelled recently. You are concerned that he is turning to alcohol to cope with his problems and may put patient safety at risk.

You are also concerned about Dr Tina Dodd (Case 4). She is an FY2 doctor who recently failed to act appropriately to a high potassium result of 6.1 which was called through by the laboratory at 10/thin;am. She performed a venous blood gas which confirmed the result but failed to act on it. When you arrived on shift at 5/thin;pm, a nurse informed you about the previous result. You immediately performed a venous blood gas which showed the potassium was 6.7. You acted according to the hospital's hyperkalaemia protocol and the patient came to no harm. You are concerned that Tina did not manage this patient appropriately.

Key points for example 13

- You should both agree that all 4 cases are important to discuss, but you should try to discuss them in order of priority given that time is short. For example you could say, "All of the cases are important for us to discuss, perhaps we should discuss these in order of priority particularly because some involve direct concerns about patient safety."

- Patient safety is paramount. This should serve as a useful guide to identifying priority. The GMC 'Good Medical Practice' guidance is a key document which you could make reference to during the group discussion.

- Each case will generate interesting discussion. You should try to remain unbiased at all times and not to attribute blame or point the finger. You should aim to 'think outside the box.'

- **Case 1 discussion points:** This case demonstrates a lack of professional integrity and teamwork skills. The fact that he is no longer considered trustworthy could result in a difficult clinical relationship. But you need to highlight that this must not affect patient care in any way. Consider if he could have been genuinely unwell, has he behaved like this before or since, why wasn't his annual leave granted, perhaps there is a lack of doctors to cover?

- **Case 2 discussion points:** This case identifies concern for a colleague. As doctors we have a duty to our patients, but also share an interest in looking out for our colleagues. You should discuss if Dr Randan feels under pressure, or if she has difficulty with time management. Does she need support, how many other juniors are in her team? The brief clearly states that there is no concern about patient safety. But you may want to discuss what kind of jobs she is doing late in the evening, for example is she writing TTAs in preparation for the next day or is she doing bloods which should have been done hours ago?

- **Case 3 discussion points:** This case also highlights concern for a colleague – but patient safety is identified as being at risk. As per the GMC Good Medical Practice guidelines you must report this to an appropriate person of authority. In this scenario, it will be your consultant. As part of the discussions you must consider and decide if it is appropriate for one of you to speak with Dr Kays about his problems and the need for action. You may be able to offer some advice and point him in the direction of 'doctors in difficulty' services.

- **Case 4 discussion points:** This case is also of high concern due to patient safety. It is likely that details are also needed from Dr Dodd about the case: why did she not act on the reading? Have there been any other cases in which she has made errors or failed to act? Is she aware of the medical emergencies and how to manage them according to local protocols/guidance? This case will also need to be discussed with an appropriate person of authority..

- Succinctly summarise at the end of your meeting, the agreed action plan for the consultant.

Worked example 14

Information for the applicant

You are one of two GP partners who have met to discuss a breach in confidentiality by one of your receptionists.

A 15-year-old female patient recently came to see one of the salaried GPs in the practice to discuss contraception following a termination of pregnancy (TOP). The patient's aunt is a new part-time receptionist in the practice, and she later entered the computerised notes and read details of the consultation and her niece's TOP. The patient was entirely unaware of this, until her aunt confronted her about the TOP. The patient returned to the practice to complain about this incident and that her confidentiality had been breeched. She made a formal complaint and demanded that action be taken.

You are meeting today to discuss this, what action to take and how such events can be avoided in future.

Write your pre-meeting thoughts and notes below:

Information for the role player (*not* to be read by the applicant)

You are one of two GP partners who have met to discuss a breach in confidentiality by one of your receptionists.

A 15-year-old female patient recently came to see one of the salaried GPs in the practice to discuss contraception following a termination of pregnancy (TOP). The patient's aunt is a new part-time receptionist in the practice, and she later entered the computerised notes and read details of the consultation and her niece's TOP. The patient was entirely unaware of this, until her aunt confronted her about the TOP. The patient returned to the practice to complain about this incident and that her confidentiality had been breeched. She made a formal complaint and demanded that action be taken.

You are meeting today to discuss this, what action to take and how such events can be avoided in future.

You should ask questions and encourage the applicant to demonstrate knowledge of the complaints process and also management strategy for this situation. Identify any pitfalls if appropriate and generate discussion between you.

Key points for example 14

- Identify that this is a serious issue. Confidentiality is fundamental to the doctor-patient relationship.

- You should highlight that the case itself will need to be scrutinized and a significant event analysis undertaken.

- Highlight the need to address the patient's formal complaint swiftly. Apologise early. Discuss meeting with the patient to apologise and to explore her key concerns and expectations. Demonstrate knowledge of the complaints process.

- You should discuss dismissing the receptionist.

- Discuss introducing an employment policy. Should you consider introducing a new policy not to employ staff from within the practice catchment area, or perhaps not employ family members of registered patients? Consider the feasibility of each point raised and work towards an agreed plan of action.

- Consider having restricted access to the medical computerised records for non-clinical staff. How could this be implemented, would this involve a blanket approach or individualized passwords?

- Consider widening the discussion to other members of staff within the practice for their input.

- Perhaps the topic of 'confidentiality' should be on the agenda for discussion and teaching at the next practice meeting.

Worked example 15

Information for the applicant

You work as an FY2 doctor in a rural GP surgery in a small village. You are meeting with the practice manager to discuss an aggressive patient and how the practice should deal with her behaviour.

You saw the patient, Mrs Hayward, during a consultation. She was newly registered and her notes had not been sent to the practice yet. She had presented with knee pain which she said was due to her osteoarthritis, and wanted analgesia. You prescribed her co-dydramol and asked her to return if it did not settle her pain. She seemed unkempt but was pleasant to you during the consultation.

It was a very busy surgery that morning, because the salaried doctor was unexpectedly absent due to a family death. So you were grateful for a 'quick and easy' consultation. You were conscious that the waiting room was full. Unfortunately, your printer stopped working that morning so you had to ask the patient to collect her prescription for co-dydramol from the front desk.

You later learnt from the receptionist at the practice that there was a long queue in the reception area and Mrs Hayward became very abusive to the patients queuing in front of her. She then stormed off without her prescription while swearing loudly. The receptionist highlighted to you that she was shocked by Mrs Hayward's response and felt very threatened at the time.

Write your pre-meeting thoughts and notes below:

Information for the role player (*not* to be read by the applicant)

You are the practice manager of a rural GP surgery in a small village. You have met with the FY2 doctor in your practice to discuss an aggressive patient and how the practice should deal with her behaviour.

You witnessed Mrs Hayward's abusive behaviour towards other patients queuing in-front of her. One of them was a young child who looked frightened. You went to intervene, but Mrs Hayward fled without collecting her prescription

The FY2 doctor had seen the patient just before the incident happened during a consultation and you would like to discuss the doctor's encounter with the patient. You would like to discuss how the practice should deal with this patient's behaviour. You will discuss the issue at the next practice meeting, but need to have the facts correct beforehand.

Key points for example 15

- This scenario clearly demonstrates why it is vital to read your brief very carefully. There's a lot of information in there.

- You should share your encounter with the patient openly. Don't be tempted to be influenced by the practice manager's negative experience. You can only comment on how the patient was with you during the consultation as stated in the brief.

- Nevertheless, you must take the patient's aggressive behaviour seriously. From your encounter with the patient, you don't know about her background or medical history. Could she have an underlying mental health disorder or social issues? How can you obtain more information about her? Should you call the previous GP, because the notes have not yet arrived? Should the patient be taking regular medications which she is no longer getting because she is new to the area?

- Discuss if the doctor should have taken a full medical and social history from the patient given that she was new to the practice. Discuss the time constraints and difficulties on that particular day. Should a locum have been called?

- Is there a practice policy for compassionate leave and cover? Is there a template for the first consultation with a newly registered patient? If not, should there be one?

- You could touch on when it may be appropriate to end a professional relationship with a patient, however this would be a very premature course of action in this scenario.

- One could argue that the patient was provoked due to practice issues which triggered the outburst. Who is responsible for maintenance of printers/IT callout and were they notified about the broken printer?

- From the receptionist's perspective, she clearly felt vulnerable and threatened at the front desk. Do you need 'zero tolerance' campaign posters displayed in the practice? Should a panic button be installed at the reception desk for staff? Should the police be called for such incidents?

- Consider the disruption this patient has caused and her impact on other patients and the reputation of the practice if her behaviour continues.

- Summarize your discussion and agreed plan of how to deal with this situation, and that it should be discussed again at the next practice meeting.

Worked example 16

Information for the applicant

You are a GP running the family planning clinic. The Trust wants you to change patients from one type of oral contraceptive pill to another brand which is cheaper. The hormonal constituents of both and side effect profile are exactly the same. You are in favour of this change and believe it will save the Trust money.

You are meeting with a GP colleague within the family planning clinic, who disagrees with the change. You hope to discuss the issues and reach an agreement.

Write your pre-meeting thoughts and notes below:

Information for the role player (*not* to be read by the applicant)

You are a GP working in the family planning clinic. The Trust wants you to change patients from one type of oral contraceptive pill to another brand which is cheaper. The hormonal constituents of both and side effect profile are exactly the same. You are against this change and believe that the cost of changing all the patients to the new tablet will be significant and would not save the Trust money overall.

You are meeting with a GP colleague within the family planning clinic, who agrees with the change. You hope to discuss the issues and reach an agreement.

Key points for example 16

- This case allows you to demonstrate your ability to discuss a new proposal, balance it with a colleague's views and reach an agreed decision. It can also highlight your awareness of evidence-based medicine and the need for lifelong learning.

- Consider the evidence that both drugs have the same constituents and side-effect profile. Are the mechanisms of action the same? Will patients need to be informed of different 'missed pill' rules?

- Consider it from the patients' perspective. Will they want to be changed from a drug they are happy on to another just because it is cheaper for the Trust? Will they feel bitter or complain if the new tablet does not suit them?

- Who will be responsible for recalling and changing all the patients over from the old to the new pill? What are the patient safety implications of having a blanket approach to changing everyone over to the new tablet? Should each patient be reviewed first? Will the Trust pay for the costs of all this?

- Remember, there is no right or wrong answer. The key is how you interact with your colleague, discuss the points and how you work together to reach an agreed decision.

Worked example 17

Information for the applicant

You are one of two GP partners who have met to discuss a prescription error.

An incident recently occurred which involved a patient with chronic heart failure not receiving enough diuretic medication. She subsequently became fluid overloaded and required emergency admission for pulmonary oedema. She is currently stable in hospital.

It later transpired that the patient's heart failure medication was recently up-titrated by the hospital during an out-patient clinic. A letter was sent from the doctor in the out-patient clinic informing the GP of the consultation and mentioned the change in medication. Unfortunately, the change was not picked up by Dr Harris, the GP who read the letter, and not coded or modified on the computer system. Therefore, when the repeat prescription was issued, it still was at the lower dose.

You are meeting with Dr Butler, a GP partner in your practice, to discuss this and how such errors can be avoided in future.

Write your pre-meeting thoughts and notes overleaf:

Information for the role player (*not* to be read by the applicant)

You are Dr Butler, a GP partner. You are meeting with another GP partner at your practice to discuss a prescription error.

An incident recently occurred which involved a patient with chronic heart failure not receiving enough diuretic medication. She subsequently became fluid overloaded and required emergency admission for pulmonary oedema. She is currently stable in hospital.

It later transpired that the patient's heart failure medication was recently up-titrated by the hospital during an out-patient clinic. A letter was sent from the doctor in the out-patient clinic informing the GP of the consultation and mentioned the change in medication. Unfortunately, the change was not picked up by Dr Harris, another GP who read the letter, and not coded or modified on the computer system. Therefore, when the repeat prescription was issued, it still was at the lower dose.

Key points for example 17

- This case raises several important points for discussion.

- The handover of care between secondary and primary care can be a risky transition. Both environments are busy and information can sometimes be overlooked. However, this is no excuse for compromised patient care and subsequent error.

- Is there any particular reason the GP who read the hospital's letter overlooked the change in medication? Consider what to do about all the other letters this GP has read. Should they be rechecked for any potentially missed action points?

- Should the hospital doctor have placed more emphasis on the change in medication (perhaps written in capital letters or have a separate section for changes to medications)? Was the patient told about the change in dose? Did she realize she had been given the old dose?

- Consider the patient's perspective. An apology must be made to the patient. Has she lost faith in the system? Will she want to have her future care provided by this hospital and your GP surgery? Should the patient be counselled and educated about her drugs so that she feels more empowered?

- A significant event analysis should be performed for this case.

- Consider what systems could be introduced to stop this from happening again and how they could be implemented.

- Summarise your discussion and action points.

Worked example 18

Information for the applicant

You are an FY2 doctor on a busy surgical rotation. You arrange to meet for lunch with an FY2 colleague, Dr Samantha Jones, whom you noted to be low in mood. You hope to discuss this with her.

You noted that Samantha has been very withdrawn and detached lately. She has started to arrive late for the morning ward rounds. Recently Samantha made an error by putting the wrong patient's details on a referral letter. Lucky it was swiftly detected because the referral was regarding a testicular lump, but a female patient's details had been mistakenly entered. She appears very tired all the time and low in mood. A colleague mentioned to you that he saw Samantha crying in the mess last week.

Write your pre-meeting thoughts and notes below:

Information for the role player (*not* to be read by the applicant)

You are Dr Samantha Jones, an FY2 in a busy surgical rotation. Your colleague has arranged to meet for lunch with you. You do not know if this is for a particular reason, or that your colleague wants to discuss any issues with you.

You have recently been feeling low in mood due to relationship difficulties. You discovered that you are pregnant last week. You want to keep the baby. You have not had any self-harm or suicidal ideations. But you are struggling to concentrate at work. You feel that some time off work would help but you know the team is very busy and organising leave is difficult.

You should respond openly or defensively depending on how the applicant approaches the subject. You should only offer information if asked about it. You may cry if you feel comfortable with the applicant.

Key points for example 18

- Handling colleagues is a common theme in the GPST entry process.

- Approach the subject with care. Bear in mind that you are only meeting for lunch and that your colleague is not expecting the Spanish Inquisition.

- Could she have any underlying personal, emotional or financial problems? Is she depressed? Does she need medical input from her own GP?

- Remember, a difficult or withdrawn doctor is often a doctor in difficulty.

- Perhaps she has professional worries. Does she feel able to do the job, is she being overworked, does she feel competent enough?

- Consider if there are any safety issues which may need addressing urgently.

- Who and how should a discussion take place with this GP about the concerns raised? Should it be a one-to-one chat or a formal meeting?

- Consider how her performance could be monitored.

- Discuss the option of her taking time off to help. Does she feel this would help? If so, think about how it could be organised.

- Remember, you can offer support, but highlight the need to involve a senior.

Worked example 19

Information for the applicant

You are an FY2 doctor in a hospital. You have been asked to discuss with a colleague why junior doctors' attendance at a morning educational lecture has been poor. It occurs weekly from 8-9 am. You have been asked to think of possible solutions and feedback to the postgraduate education co-ordinator.

Write your pre-meeting thoughts and notes below:

Information for the role player (*not* to be read by the applicant)

You are an FY2 doctor in a hospital. You have been asked to discuss with a colleague why junior doctors' attendance at a morning educational lecture has been poor. It occurs weekly from 8-9 am.. You have been asked to think of possible solutions and feedback to the postgraduate education co-ordinator.

Note: the applicant and role player briefs are the same.

You should ask questions and generate discussion.

Key points for example 19

- Consider reasons why attendance is poor and the solutions.

- Advertising: are people aware of these sessions? Should they be advertised in the mess or highlighted in the induction programme?

- Timing: are they held too early, do they clash with preparation for the morning ward round? Should they be moved to a lunchtime session?

- Topics: have the topics been interesting, stimulating or relevant to the doctors' learning needs? Should the junior doctors suggest potential topics, so that the teaching is tailored to the requests?

- Mandatory: Perhaps the session should be incorporated into mandatory teaching. Consider the issues around having another hour of mandatory teaching per week. Would it be bleep-free, would the wards and seniors allow time away from the ward?

- You could discuss setting up a questionnaire or survey to canvas opinions about this teaching session. This would give a more accurate picture and help the postgraduate education co-ordinator make an informed decision about what to do.

Worked example 20

Information for the applicant

You are a GP in a meeting with the practice manager. The practice has recently received a £1 000 donation from a patient. The staff at the practice have short-listed 4 options for how the money should be spent

1. *To buy equipment for the consultation rooms. For example, you are aware that there is only one otoscope and fundoscope in the practice. Other small, but necessary, items are also required in all of the consultation rooms, such as tendon hammers and pen torches.*

2. *To create and publish a newsletter for the practice to highlight the achievements to date and use is as a health promotion tool. There are only enough funds to publish one bewsletter.*

3. *To fund a practice event. For example, a staff away-day which would involve team building exercises like paint-balling, or the next Christmas dinner.*

4. *To renovate the practice. The waiting area is particularly run-down. It needs painting and some new furniture to give it a fresh and inviting atmosphere which would benefit the patients and staff.*

You are meeting to discuss the options and decide which option to go for.

Write your pre-meeting thoughts and notes below:

Information for the role player (*not* to be read by the applicant)

You are the practice manager in a meeting with a GP. The practice has recently received a £1 000 donation from a patient. The staff at the practice have short-listed 4 options for how the money should be spent

1. *To buy equipment for the consultation rooms. For example, you are aware that there is only one otoscope and fundoscope in the practice. Other small, but necessary, items are also required in all of the consultation rooms, such as tendon hammers and pen torches.*

2. *To create and publish a newsletter for the practice to highlight the achievements to date and use is as a health promotion tool. There are only enough funds to publish one newsletter.*

3. *To fund a practice event. For example, a staff away-day which would involve team building exercises like paint-balling, or the next Christmas dinner.*

4. *To renovate the practice. The waiting area is particularly run-down. It needs painting and some new furniture to give it a fresh and inviting atmosphere which would benefit the patients and staff.*

You are meeting to discuss the options and decide which option to go for.

Note: the applicant and role player brief are the same for this scenario.

Key points practice example 20

- This case allows discussion of social, professional, educational and ethical principles.

- Do not be overly dismissive of any one idea in particular. You should allow the practice manager to share her thoughts. Invite her to share the thoughts of other team members if she is aware of them, and be respectful towards their views.

- Before deciding what to do with the sum of money, you should consider who it came from and why was it donated? Is there ulterior motive behind the donation? It is a sizeable sum, so you should consider if the practice is allowed to accept the donation.

- Renovate the practice: this idea allows the donation to be invested in both the practice and patients. Is there any supporting evidence that this work needs to be done, for example have any patients complained or was it mentioned in previous patient surveys? Consider if £1000 worth of paint and furniture is a lot? Perhaps the donation could be split and some spent on paint and some on another idea.

- Staff away-day / Christmas dinner: consider the advantages and disadvantages of this idea. The other ideas offer some form of 'investment' in the practice, whereas this idea appears more frivolous with no benefit to patients. How would the practice be perceived, would it be considered professional, would patients or organisation donate money in the future?

- Equipment for practice: this would offer benefit to patients and the clinicians using the equipment. Does the practice need more than one otoscope or fundoscope, how much demand is there for it on a regular basis? Consider if it would be helpful to order smaller items, such as tendon hammers and pen torches, so that each consultation room is fully equipped. It may mean less time looking around for one when needed, so a swifter consultation and less delay in seeing other patients.

- Print a practice newsletter: this is an interesting and innovative idea; consider its advantages and disadvantages. How many pages would it be: doubled sided A4, double sided A3 folded in half, etc? What information would be included in the newsletter? Who would be the target audience? Which health promotion topics would be included? Is doing it as a 'one-off' project worthwhile?

12 Written prioritization exercise

Annabelle Macgregor

Basis and format of the WPE

A career as a GP is diverse and challenging and without doubt all GPs have days when they feel overwhelmed with the volume of work and short of free time. In order to succeed as a GP, give the best care to our patients and prevent emotional stress or disillusionment in the long term, we all need strategies and personal skills to help us cope with multiple demands on our time. In essence, the written prioritization exercise is designed to test these abilities. You need to show that you can remain calm, think logically, be organized and efficient. You also need to demonstrate your ability to delegate when appropriate, while retaining responsibility for your actions and that you are aware that your own personal needs are important and can affect your performance at work.

The prioritization exercise is the only written exercise of the stage 3 selection centre. It is marked solely on what you have put on your answer paper. You will be given a scenario where you are either a hospital doctor or a doctor working in general practice. After the scenario, there will be five or six tasks which you have to prioritize. You will be asked to place each of the tasks in the order that you would carry them out. You will also have to give reasons for your ranking. Following this, there are usually a couple of additional questions designed to make you reflect on how you felt about the exercise overall. The assessment is timed and you usually have 20–30 minutes to complete it depending on your deanery.

What are the examiners looking for?

The scoring is based on the GP NPS and in order to do well it is important to be familiar with the skills that are being evaluated. The prioritization exercise is entirely written and therefore it is vital to show that you possess these abilities through your written answers. This section sets out how to demonstrate these skills in this assessment.

Clinical knowledge and expertise: written prioritization exercise

The fact that you have made it this far in the selection process is because you showed in stage 2 that you have enough clinical knowledge to potentially train as a GP. Stage 3 is much more concerned with assessing your personal skills. Therefore, your focus in this exercise should not be solely concerned with demonstrating your clinical acumen. It is of course important however, to show you have the knowledge to act safely. For example, writing discharge summaries before going to see a patient with central crushing chest pain is difficult to justify in any circumstances.

For this exercise, the examiners want you to demonstrate a safe approach based on your clinical knowledge. For example, all emergencies should be dealt with first. If you are given two or more stems which are emergencies, then you could demonstrate your knowledge of 'ABC' and base your decisions on those that deal with 'airway' problems first, then 'breathing' and then 'circulation.' However, all answers will depend largely on the given scenario and context. So always read the question very carefully and apply your knowledge accordingly.

Empathy and sensitivity: written prioritization exercise

The ability to understand other points of view and empathize with people is an essential skill for a GP. This skill can be more difficult to demonstrate in a written exercise than the other personal skills. Nevertheless, it is important to show that you respect other perspectives, can understand patients' concerns and expectations, especially when they are different to your own. You should demonstrate that you are a supportive member of the team and respect the views of the multidisciplinary team.

Communication skills: written prioritization exercise

Written communication is equally important for communication with colleagues and in the medicolegal climate in which we work. For the purposes of the GP entry process, your written communication skills will be directly tested in the stage 3 written prioritization exercise. You will need to demonstrate:

- Clear expression of written thought – must be legible (obviously!), well reasoned and systematic.
- Good communication with others, particularly in difficult situations (i.e. MDT, patients), i.e. know how you delegate and thank others for helping.
- Varied vocabulary and appropriate use of language.
- Aim to use the first person tense and use your natural writing style – makes your answer more personable and will help the assessor gain an idea of your personality. A third person response with little expression of emotion is unlikely to help.
- Reflect clearly on the exercise and what you have learnt from it.

The last two points will be continuously required in your subsequent GP training within the e-portfolio and for appraisals/ revalidation. It is an essential skill worth learning early so practise, practise and practise.

You could use bullet points if you prefer, but many applicants find it easier to express their thoughts better in continuous prose. Practise using both methods and decide which suits you best. Remember that you must keep a close eye on the clock. It is easy to get carried away in this exercise and lose track of the remaining time. This will disadvantage you because there are valuable marks at the end of the exercise when reflecting on what you learnt.

Conceptual thinking and problem solving: written prioritization exercise

This exercise is very good at assessing your conceptual thinking and problem solving skills. Often, the scenario you are given contains little detailed information. This is deliberate. It attempts to get you thinking outside the box and not to take things at 'face value'. You should state that you would ask for more details, but often even in reality we do not have many details when attending to a patient, for example in an emergency. So you need to formulate a management plan based on the information you have. You will need to show that you have considered other possibilities. The examiner will want you to have at least thought of the best- and worst-case scenario and have thought about how you may deal with each if it were the case.

The scenario is unlikely to be straightforward. In our daily practice we often have to manage challenging situations, which usually involve several difficult tasks compounded by limited time and resources, such as manpower. For example, consider a typical surgical on-call shift with numerous discharge summaries to complete, some post-op reviews, a very sick patient who you are attending and incessant sounding of your bleep. This situation is compounded by your senior being in theatre, and another bleep sounding about a very sick patient needing your review. What would you do first? How would you manage the tasks?

You need to show that you can judge what is important from the information you have. The examiner will want you to demonstrate your ability to think beyond the apparent facts and recognize that there may be a number of solutions to the problem. The information you are given regarding each task is often limited and you need to show the ability to adapt to be flexible in your approach and can adapt to changing circumstances. It is also a chance to show you are organized both with your time and resources and are able to delegate.

Coping with pressure: written prioritization exercise

Coping with pressure in this exercise can be demonstrated by recognizing your limitations, seeking help from colleagues, acknowledging the impact of your actions on others, recognizing your own needs to maintain a work–life balance and implementing your coping strategies. Attempting to be a superhero by taking on all the tasks might seem to be a good way to demonstrate your skills, but it is unlikely you would be able to carry them all out effectively. It is vital to show that you recognize this and understand the importance of other's contributions, are able to share the load and work in a team.

Your management of work–life balance and recognition of your personal needs can be easily assessed in this exercise. Being a GP is of course stressful and you need to show you have the ability to recognize the impact of this on your own life and that you have strategies to deal with it and make time to look after yourself. Providing patient safety is not put at risk, you would not be marked down for prioritizing a personal situation above a clinical situation. However, you must write clear justification for your ranking.

Organization and planning: written prioritization exercise

When answering any question which assesses your ability to prioritize, you must always demonstrate that you are a safe doctor and not put your patients at risk. In our role as doctors, it is not possible to do everything by yourself. Therefore, you must also demonstrate that you can recognize when to ask for help from others, how to delegate and share tasks with your team. Some applicants do not realize that in this exercise you are allowed to utilize and share jobs with other team members around, but you must do so safely. You should aim to demonstrate to who, how and why you would delegate a particular task and how that helps. You should bear in mind that you would not want to be seen as shirking responsibility.

In your answer try to explain what you would do in reality. For example, if you were attending to a sick patient you would kindly ask a nurse to make an emergency call, rather than leave the patient to make the call yourself. Be systematic in your planning and reasoning.

Managing others and team involvement: written prioritization exercise

It is essential that you can show that you can work as part of a team and you respect the contributions of others. Therefore you need to show the ability to delegate work appropriately while continuing to recognize your own responsibilities.

In order to prioritize safely and effectively, you must have an awareness of each team member's role. You could demonstrate this skill to the examiner by highlighting in your justification why you delegated a particular task to a particular colleague rather than another available colleague.

Professional integrity: written prioritization exercise

It is important that you take responsibility for your actions and demonstrate that you respect other people's roles and abilities. It is also important that you help generate a safe atmosphere. You are personally accountable for your actions and must always be prepared to justify your decisions and actions.

Learning and personal development: written prioritization exercise

You can show that you have the commitment to personal development by showing that you understand the importance of reflecting on experiences and that you are able to use this knowledge to continue to learn.

The reflective question carries marks. So pace yourself and work quickly, because time is very tight for this exercise.

How to prioritize

The first important point is that it is essential to recognize that there are no absolute right or wrong answers in this exercise in terms of how you rank the tasks. There are many more marks available for the reasons behind the order you have put the tasks in than the order itself so spend most time on this. However, there are some sensible general rules about prioritizing tasks.

In general, the tasks will be a combination of:

- Clinical tasks involving patients that may be urgent or not so urgent. For example, a patient on the ward with shortness of breath or a patient on the telephone with chest pain.
- Other clinical tasks involving patient care. For example, writing referral letters or prescriptions.
- Tasks relating to your work that are not patient related. For example, audit projects, management issues or teaching.
- Personal tasks, for example, eating lunch, phoning your mother or booking a holiday.

It sounds obvious, but the first rule is to prioritize the tasks in terms of importance and urgency. Safety is paramount and, if there is any task where staff, patients or other people's safety is at risk, it is vital it is dealt with swiftly.

Look for any urgent clincial problems as these should be addressed immediately. These may involve patients with symptoms or signs of serious illness or investigations which suggest that immediate treatment may be required or, for example, a patient in pain. It also includes patients who could potentially deteriorate quickly.

The information you are given is often limited so try to think widely about what the scenario might be suggesting in deciding whether it is urgent. A simple example is a diabetic patient with hyperglycaemia. They may be well and only need a change in their long-term medication, but without further information you cannot exclude diabetic ketoacidosis and therefore you need to assume it is an urgent problem until you have been able to ascertain other information. Once you have this information your priority in dealing with this case might become less urgent.

After dealing with urgent cases, in general, clinical patient-related tasks should be dealt with before other tasks. However, remember this does not always have to be the case. So, for example, there may be deadlines you have to adhere to or other professionals may be involved in the task and it may not be appropriate to keep them waiting. In these situations, non-clinical tasks may need to be done before particular clinical tasks.

It is also important to remember your own personal needs and not automatically put these last. Worrying about an issue outside work can be very distracting and affect the clinical care you provide and sometimes a quick phone call can set your mind at rest.

If you are struggling with placing certain tasks, think about the potential outcomes of delaying the task. Also consider how long it would take you to carry out the task, because some tasks can be sorted out very quickly and therefore are better placed above a task which might take you some time.

Don't try to do everything yourself or you will fail! Always ask yourself what other help do I have available, are there other clinical staff who could see a patient for example, can the administration staff ease your workload by giving you results or further information to help you prioritize. Be aware that when you delegate you need to ensure that the person to whom you give the task has the appropiate qualifications and expertise for that task. You also need to remember that when you delegate you don't absolve yourself of all responsibility, so make sure you check the outcome at some point and find out if there is anything left for you to do.

Reflecting on the exercise

In general, there will always be a couple of questions at the end which allow you to reflect on the exercise overall. Questions might include:

- Which task did you find hardest to prioritize and why?
- What did you feel went well?
- What have you found difficult about this exercise?

- What have you learnt from the exercise?
- What might you do differently next time?

Reflection is a process we often do subconsciously and sometimes more overtly, for example debriefing after a difficult cardiac arrest. Reflecting on your own practice is vital to assess your continued learning needs, and important both as a trainee and a fully-fledged GP. It forms a key part of demonstrating your ability and willingness to learn from experience. It is an essential process for continuing to develop and improve your practice. Even when everything went well, there is usually room for some improvement.

The key to answering these questions is to be open and honest. There is little value trying to learn a set answer because you never know how you will feel on the day with the particular tasks you are set. It is likely to be a challenging exercise. We all have to prioritize tasks on a daily basis, but do we make the right decisions and how could we do better?

Top 10 tips for the day

1. There is no doubt that the key to success in this exercise is to familiarize yourself with the criteria that you are being asked to demonstrate and practise, practise, practise. Think about your day-to-day work and how you prioritize tasks in practice. Consider how you would rank and justify in writing your actions.

2. Before your assessment, check with your deanery how much time you have to complete the exercise and practise within this time allocation. The time will always be very limited and you need to be sure you are able to complete it all, including the reflective exercise, to do well.

3. On the day, take a watch with you. Have a plan for how you are going to use your time and stick to it rigidly. If you have time at the end you can always add more, but make sure you answer all the parts of the assessment.

4. Do not run out of time. I allowed 5 minutes to read through the exercise and think about it before starting writing and even then time was tight.

5. When you are reading the exercise make a particular note of who you are and where you are (e.g. SHO in A&E, FY2 in general practice, etc.). Start thinking about what other help is potentially available to you and means of communication other than face to face that may save you time, e.g. email, telephone consultations, etc.

6. Read through all the tasks before starting and make a decision about ranking and then stick to it. There are many more points to be gained in justifying your decisions and this is where you should spend more time.

7. Think about how best to convey the information. Some people find writing in bullet points is the quickest and helps you to order your points.

8. Even though you need to write fast, be legible. Otherwise it is all a waste of time. Try not to have lots of crossings out by making decisions about what you are going to write before committing it to the answer paper.

9. Do not forget to have some time at the end for the reflective section, it is important.

10. Finally stay calm: this exercise is about showing you can cope with pressure.

Worked example 1

You are a GP and have just come to the end of a busy afternoon surgery.

The tasks below need to be done and must be prioritized for action, which involves three stages:

    1. Rank each task in the order you intend to deal with it.
    2. Justify your ranking decisions.
    3. Comment on interesting or challenging issues encountered within this exercise.

Use the answer sheet to rank the highest priority task in the first box and work down until you have ranked the task of least priority. Enter your justification and comments relating to each task respectively on the answer sheet.

You have 30 minutes in total for this exercise. Do not write for the first 5 minutes. You should read the tasks and challenge. You will be instructed when you can start writing.

You will have 20 minutes to rank the tasks and justify your ranking.

You will have 5 minutes to complete the reflection task.

Tasks to be ranked:
A. The receptionist comes to give you a message that Mrs Carr, a patient, would like to speak to you.
B. The practice manager knocks on the door wanting to discuss QOF (quality and outcomes framework) targets.
C. One of the practice nurses rings saying she needs your help with a patient, she is doing an immunization clinic.
D. You notice you have a message on your mobile phone asking you to ring your son's nursery.
E. From your room you can hear a patient shouting in reception. He is upset about the wait to be seen by you.

Reflection question: Which task did you find most difficult to prioritize?

Enter your answer to example 1 below

Rank:

Rank:

Rank:

Rank:

Rank:

Reflection:

Prioritizing example 1 – a suggested approach

Before reading through this, remember there is no exact right answer.

Look for any urgent clinical issues or safety issues and put these at the top. In this example, there are two tasks which should be done urgently. Option E raises concern about safety for other members of staff and for patients in the waiting room. Option C is less obvious because you have very little information, but this could be a patient having an anaphylactic reaction to an immunization.

In trying to prioritize these two tasks, think about what help you have available. In a general practice setting, there will be other clinical staff (such as partners, salaried GPs, trainees, practice nurses, HCAs), administrative/clinical staff (such as receptionists, secretaries), the practice manager and other staff (e.g. midwives, counsellors, health visitors, etc.). Think about their roles and qualifications as to how best they might be able to help you. In this case, there may be other clinical staff free to assist the nurse while you go to reception, but option C is a potentially life-threatening situation and so you should do it yourself, and avoid wasting time by looking for someone to delegate this task to. The practice manager is at your door and therefore it would appear to make sense that you delegate for the practice manager to go and help with the problem at reception, while you deal with the clinical case.

Of the three tasks left, you have one that is patient related, another patient unrelated (QOF targets) and one personal. It is tempting to put the clinical task next, however it is highly likely that the call from the nursery will be worrying you and could distract you. Delaying the task in option D, could make it difficult for you to concentrate until you have established what the call was about. Therefore, this could be done next.

The fourth task would be option A to ring the patient. This is a difficult task to prioritize as there is very little information, but there is currently nothing suggesting it is an emergency. Before you get to do this task, think about whether there is anything you can do to help you prioritize further. For example, one of the HCAs or nurses could ring her to get more information to decide how urgent it is. A receptionist or administrative staff could check who saw the patient last as, if it was recently, it might be more appropriate that that person rang them if they were available.

Talking to the practice manager would come last in this case, although it is important to stress that good communication and cooperation is essential for running a successful and effective service. Think about other ways you could communicate with the practice manager.

Suggested answer to worked example 1

Ranking: CEDAB

Rank 1: C

I would go to the nurse first. I know she is doing an immunization clinic and in the absence of further information I have to assume there may be an urgent clinical problem, such as anaphylaxis. I would apologise to the practice manager but I am sure he understands that urgent clinical problems come first. Although there may be other clinical staff free to go to this patient I think that given the potential urgency I would go there immediately to assist the nurse before looking for other staff. If when I got there the patient needed urgent clinical attention I would administer this and stay with the patient until they were stable. I would ask the receptionist to call a 999 ambulance while I continue to treat the patient. I may well need some assistance and ask if anyone was free to find out if there were any other clinical staff free. Teamwork is essential for providing optimal clinical care.

If the problem was less clinically urgent and there was another doctor free then I would ask if they were able to deal with it. If no one was free and the issue was something that could not be dealt with very quickly, I would apologise to the patient for not being able to deal with the problem immediately and explain to the patient that if she wanted to wait I would see her when I have sorted out any other urgent problems, or that I would be happy to book her an appointment to see her in a surgery or a telephone appointment if that is appropriate.

Anaphylaxis is an uncommon and frightening event in a GP surgery and potentially very stressful for all those concerned. When I was able to, I would talk to the nurse involved to ensure she was OK and suggest having a debriefing at a time convenient for all those involved so we could all discuss how we dealt with this emergency.

Rank 2: E

An angry patient is potentially an issue of safety for other patients in reception and staff and it is important to keep everyone safe, but also to support staff in this difficult situation. The practice manager is at my door, so I would apologise for not being able to talk immediately and see if he would be able to go to reception to help, while I saw the patient with the practice nurse. I would suggest to the practice manager that it might be pertinent to take the patient to a private room to speak to him, while ensuring everyone remains safe.

As soon as I was free after seeing the patient from the immunization clinic, I would go to reception. I would apologise to the patient and explain that there has been an urgent clinical issue which prevented me seeing him sooner.

I would see him now as he may simply be angry because of the wait or there may be a more urgent problem going on, which is making him behave differently from normal. He might be in pain, it may be that he is confused or has mental health problems or withdrawing from alcohol or drugs, for example. There is the potential that he may become violent and therefore it would be important to move him away from the waiting room while ensuring I maintain my own safety and that of other people around. Dealing with angry patients can be upsetting and alarming for staff involved and I would ensure that when I had seen the patient I would check that the staff involved were alright.

Rank 3: D

After dealing with the urgent clinical problems, I would phone the nursery as I do not know the reason they wanted to contact me. If I do not do this now it is likely to play on my mind and affect my ability to work. In order to be competent and to provide the best care for my patients, it is very important that I am not distracted by personal worries. It may be that something has happened that I need to deal with immediately or it may just be that they wanted to let me know something routine, but if I do not find out I know it will divert my attention and affect my clinical care. If it is something urgent, for example my son has had an accident, I may need to leave work immediately. If this is the case I would ensure that my clinical work is covered by available colleagues and when I return I would liaise with them to check whether there was anything I needed to follow up from this.

Rank 4: A

In the absence of further information I would phone Mrs Carr now. While I am dealing with the urgent problems I would see whether any staff were free to ring her to find out a bit more information to help me prioritize. There may be other clinical staff free who were available to speak to her before I could. I would also ask reception to check her notes to see when she was last seen and by whom as it might be more appropriate that they rang her if they were available now. If there is no one free I would ring her when I am free. I would familiarize myself with her notes before I rang her. When I speak to her, I would apologise for the delay in speaking to her.

Rank 5: B

Good communication with the practice manager is obviously very important for the running of a good and successful practice. However, I am sure the practice manager understands that clinical care often has to take priority. If he has to leave before I am free to talk to him I would offer to ring him later on his mobile. However, it may be more appropriate to meet with all the clinical staff at the practice as they are all involved in QOF and I would suggest this to him. If this is the case, it might be a good idea for him to email everyone about the issues to be discussed beforehand so they have an opportunity to consider them.

Reflective question: Which task did you find most difficult to prioritize?

I found it most difficult to prioritize the practice manager wanting to talk with me. I felt uncomfortable that I had to keep a colleague waiting. However, I had to prioritize the situations before me based on clinical urgency first, and then address a task which would have distracted me and potentially impaired my ability to fully concentrate and complete another task unless I telephoned my child's nursery.

I worried that it may show a lack of respect towards the practice manager. So I would explain the situation and apologise to the practice manager. I would also arrange a suitable time to meet with the practice manager to discuss any issues.

Worked example 2

You are a surgical Foundation Year 2 doctor on call for the night. You have just taken hand-over and have the following tasks to do.

A. *Mr Ross, a GP referral with suspected bowel obstruction is waiting to be seen. His observations are apparently stable.*
B. *There are three drug charts that need rewriting*
C. *Mr Singh's catheter is blocked.*
D. *The ward sister bleeps you. Mrs Cross, who had a laparotomy 3 days ago, has chest pain.*
E. *You have to finish writing your job application. It needs to be handed in tomorrow morning.*

Reflective question: Which task would you do differently next time?

Use the answer sheet overleaf to rank the highest priority task in the first box and work down until you have ranked the task of least priority. Enter your justification and comments relating to each task respectively on the answer sheet.

Enter your answer to example 2 below

Rank:

Rank:

Rank:

Rank:

Rank:

Reflection:

Suggested answer to worked example 2

Ranking: DCABE

Rank 1: D

- Patient care is my first priority and this is a potentially urgent clinical problem. She has recently had surgery and the cause of her pain could be a PE or an MI.
- I would ask the ward sister if anyone was available to do some observations on the patient and an ECG and give her some oxygen and let her know I am on my way immediately. Effective teamwork is essential for good clinical care.
- It may be that there are other doctors available to assist me and when I arrive on the ward I would see if there were any ward staff available to contact them.
- I would assess, investigate and treat the patient as appropriate and would stay with her until she is stable or other help has arrived and I am no longer required.

Rank 2: C

- Although this is not an urgent clinical problem, if the catheter has been blocked for some time the patient may be in significant pain and therefore I should prioritize this task.
- I would ring the ward to find out some more information such as the patients medical background, the reason for the catheter and how long it has been blocked.

- The catheter may just need flushing and while on the phone to the ward I would ask if there was a nurse or healthcare assistant to do this and let me know the outcome.
- If the catheter needs reinserting, I would see if anyone else on the ward is available and qualified to do this. As I am quite busy I could also speak to the site practitioner who may know of someone who is able to go and catheterize the patient. If no one else is available and the patient is in pain I would go and resite the catheter now.

Rank 3: A

- As soon as possible, I would ring A&E to see if the patient is still stable and that there is no change in his observations.
- If he has become unstable I would go and see him immediately.
- Otherwise I would ask that A&E keep him nil by mouth (NBM) and see if anyone was free to insert a cannula, take some bloods, start some fluids and give him some analgesia and I will see him after I have recatheterized Mr Singh.
- I would also ask the nurse in A&E to contact my registrar and SHO (if I have one) to see if they are available to see the patient before I am free.
- If one of my colleagues sees the patient I would liaise with them afterwards to discuss the plan and to see whether there was anything further I needed to do.

Rank 4: B

- In the absence of further information, it is difficult to know how urgent this task is. It may be that all the drugs on the chart have already been given that night and the next drugs are in the morning or it may be more important I carry this out quickly, for example if there is a patient needing analgesia or a patient who is NBM requiring fluids.
- Therefore, I would first check with the ward staff as to the medication that needs writing up.
- If it is required imminently, I would ask the ward staff whether there is anyone free who could bring me the drug charts, with the patient's notes, to wherever I currently am, so I can rewrite them. If this is not possible because the ward is busy I would try to get to the ward as soon as I had seen the patients that needed to be seen.

Rank 5: E

- For the progression of my career, it is important that I ensure my job application is handed in on time. I would normally not leave something this important to the last minute and it is likely to play on my mind and affect my clinical care if I am unable to do it.
- However I have only just started my shift and the clinical work is currently more urgent. I would therefore deal with this once I had dealt with the other tasks.
- Reflective question: Which task would you do differently next time?
- I found tasks A and C the most difficult to prioritize and feel that maybe I should have assessed the patient with bowel obstruction before changing Mr Singh's catheter.
- In the absence of further information it was difficult to know the urgency of each task. Although the patient with suspected bowel obstruction was stable, he had the potential to deteriorate and might need fluids, analgesia and antibiotics as soon as possible. The patient in need of a new catheter might be in pain from retention and I would obviously want to act more quickly if this was the case.
- I think this situation demonstrates the importance of working as a team and delegating work where appropriate to ensure effective clinical care.

Worked example 3

You are an ST1 in A&E. Rank the tasks below and justify your ranking.

A. The biochemistry lab rings to say that Mrs Winters' potassium is 6.9. She is waiting to be seen by the on-call medical team.

B. The ward clerk informs you that security would like you to move your motorbike.

C. The daughter of Mr Joshi would like to see you. Mr Joshi was brought in 1 hour ago in cardiac arrest and it was not possible to resuscitate him.

D. The A&E secretary comes to remind you that you need to complete a police statement for a patient you saw a few months ago. It is due in 2 days.

E. *One of the nurses asks you to review Miss Jonas. She is a surgical referral with biliary colic and is in pain. The surgical team are unable to see her currently.*

Reflective question: Which task did you find easiest to prioritize?

Use the answer sheet overleaf to rank the highest priority task in the first box and work down until you have ranked the task of least priority. Enter your justification and comments relating to each task respectively on the answer sheet.

Enter your answer to example 3 below

Rank:

Rank:

Rank:

Rank:

Rank:

Reflection:

Suggested answer to worked example 3

Ranking: AEBCD

Rank 1: A

This is potentially an urgent clinical problem and I would address this first. I would go and assess this patient now. I would take a history and also examine the patient to see if I could determine the cause. I would ask if there is a phlebotomist available to repeat the U and E's and whether there is a nurse or HCA available to do an ECG. I would start any immediate treatment as required and I would then ring the medical registrar to let them know about the result and the action I have taken. I would ensure she was closely monitored and would review her until the medical team are free to see her. When they arrived to see her I would make sure I was available to handover to them as this is very important for good clinical care.

Rank 2: E

Biliary colic is not a really urgent clinical problem but the patient is in pain and I would therefore see this patient as soon as I feel the patient with hyperkalaemia is stable. I would apologise for the patient for not being able to see her immediately and explain that this was because I was dealing with an urgent clinical problem. I would prescribe her adequate analgesia and ensure she is stable and that she is able to wait for the surgeons. I would explain to her that the surgeons are currently unable to see her as they are dealing with another urgent problem, but until they arc free we would continue to monitor her and ensure her pain is under control. I would ask the nurse looking after her to do regular observation readings and to let me know if they are changing or if her pain is not under control.

Rank 3: B

In the absence of further information, it is difficult to know how urgent this task is. My motorbike may for example be parked in the wrong space or it may be blocking somewhere important, for example an ambulance entrance. It is obviously important I move it, but if it is blocking somewhere important I would first see if there was any other doctor available to see the urgent clinical cases, if this was not the case I would give the keys to a member of staff who was able to move it to a more appropriate place while I continued with my clinical work.

Rank 4: C

An important part of my clinical role involves seeing relatives of patients and answering their questions and keeping them informed. It is therefore important I go and speak to Mr Joshi's daughter as soon as possible. However, the urgent clinical tasks would take priority over this. I would first check whether there was anyone else involved in the resuscitation who would be free to talk to them before I could. If this is not the case I would ask someone to apologise to them and explain that I am involved in an emergency, but I will see them as soon as possible. It is important when I do go to see them that I am able to give them as much time as they need and therefore need to deal with the urgent clinical times first. When I first see them I would apologise to them for the delay.

Rank 5: D

It is important to complete police statements in good time and allow the secretaries sufficient time to type them. I would therefore like to complete it today once I have completed the other tasks. I would ask the secretary if she would be able to get me a copy of the patient's notes to allow me to complete this task more quickly.

Reflective question: Which task did you find easiest to prioritize?

In the absence of further information, I felt that the patient with hyperkalaemia had to be dealt with first. This is potentially a clinically urgent problem and she has the potential to deteriorate. Patient safety and clinical care must always be my first priority and it is important that I ensure the patient is stable before I deal with other tasks.

Worked example 4

You are a junior doctor in a general practice setting. You have just finished a busy morning surgery. Rank the tasks below and justify your ranking.

> A. Mrs Brown is expecting you to ring her now with her blood results. Her results are normal.

B. *The receptionist lets you know there is a mother in reception. She has no appointment but would like her child seen – he has a rash and fever.*

C. *Mr Young is on the phone – he is experiencing chest pain and is enquiring what he should do.*

D. *You need to book a restaurant for tonight – it is your partner's birthday.*

E. *Your GP supervisor is waiting for you for a tutorial.*

Reflective question: What have you learnt from this exercise?

Use the answer sheet overleaf to rank the highest priority task in the first box and work down until you have ranked the task of least priority. Enter your justification and comments relating to each task respectively on the answer sheet.

Enter your answer to example 4 below

Rank:

Rank:

Rank:

Rank:

Rank:

Reflection:

Suggested answer to worked example 4

Ranking: CBADE

Rank 1: C

In the absence of further clinical information, I have to assume that Mr Young's chest pain could be caused by a cardiac problem. It is unlikely that I would be able to confidently exclude an acute coronary event over the phone and it is likely he would need further investigation, in particular an ECG. I would therefore ask the receptionist to let Mr Young know that I feel he needs to go to A&E by ambulance and ask the receptionist to call the ambulance for him. I would afterwards check with the receptionist to ensure this happened.

Rank 2: B

This is potentially a clinically urgent problem and I would see the child immediately. The child may simply have a viral illness, but potentially this could be, for example, meningococcal sepsis. I would therefore assess the child. I know that my supervisor is waiting for me and if I was concerned about the child I would call them for assistance and ask the receptionist to call an ambulance. If I felt the child did have significant sepsis, I would give the child antibiotics and call an ambulance.

Rank 3: A

Mrs Brown is waiting for me to call her. Even though I know her results are normal she is likely to be worrying about them. While I am dealing with the urgent clinical problems I could see if anyone else was available to ring her and let her know. If this was the case I would check with them afterwards whether she wanted to speak to me further and would ring her when available.

Rank 4: D

This is a very quick task as it would only involve a short phone call and I would therefore do it next. I think having a good balance between my work and my home life is very important in order to succeed and it is important that I do not let my work life overshadow my personal relationships.

Rank 5: E

> Attending tutorials and teaching sessions is very important personal development and for maintaining and improving my clinical effectiveness and abilities. However, urgent clinical issues will have to come before this. I would apologise to my supervisor and if I am very delayed would try and arrange another date for this session.

Reflective question: What have you learnt from this exercise?

Although it is important to deal with tasks I feel are clinically urgent quickly and effectively I always need to keep in mind and respect other people's perspectives. In this exercise, I knew Mrs Brown's results were normal and therefore from a clinical point of view this task was not particularly urgent. However, I recognize that waiting for test results can be very stressful and it was important that I set her mind at rest as soon as possible.

Worked example 5

You are a Foundation Year 2 doctor in general practice. It is 1 p.m. on a Friday afternoon. You have the following tasks to deal with:

  A. *There are a pile of results that you need to go through.*
  B. *Dr Kelly, the cardiology consultant, at your local hospital has left a message asking you to ring her about your patient Mr Kitt.*
  C. *The secretary reminds you that you need to complete the referral for a routine dermatology appointment for Mrs Charlton, whom you saw this morning.*
  D. *Mrs Lee has just arrived in reception, she is 7 weeks pregnant and has abdominal pain.*
  E. *Your brother has left a message on your phone saying your mother has been admitted to hospital.*

Reflective question: What would you do differently next time?

Use the answer sheet overleaf to rank the highest priority task in the first box and work down until you have ranked the task of least priority. Enter your justification and comments relating to each task respectively on the answer sheet.

Enter your answer to example 5 below

Rank:

Rank:

Rank:

Rank:

Rank:

Reflection:

Suggested answer to worked example 5

Ranking: DEBAC

Rank 1: D

This is potentially an urgent clinical problem. She may have an ectopic pregnancy or she may be miscarrying. In the absence of other clinical staff to see her, I would see her immediately. If I feel that she may have an ectopic I would ensure she was stable and ask reception staff to phone for an ambulance if they were able. I would inform the gynaecology team at the local hospital about her and I would explain my concerns to the patient so she is fully informed.

Rank 2: E

I would phone my brother next as otherwise I will be worrying about what has happened to my mother and this will distract me in my work. If there is an urgent problem it may be that I have to leave work. If this is the case, I would speak to one of the partners and ensure that there is adequate clinical cover for my work. When I returned to work it is important that I follow up with my colleagues the work that they did for me and discuss any follow up required.

Rank 3: B

In the absence of further information, I would phone the cardiologist now. Before this, I would ask the receptionist to check whether any other doctor is free to ring, particularly if she is known to them. I am aware that it is Friday afternoon and it may be that there is something I need to do for the patient, e.g. prescribe a new medication or there may be further information she requires to help her with her treatment and I do not want to leave it too late in the day as the weekend is coming up. Before phoning the cardiologist I would ensure I have looked through the patient's notes and medications.

Rank 4: A

Again I am aware that it is Friday afternoon and there may be results that require urgent action and it could adversely affect patient care if I leave this task too late. It is essential for patient safety that abnormal results are dealt with immediately. There may be other clinical staff who could deal with the results before I could, but if this was not the case I am aware that there are medical students waiting for me and I would ask whether they were able to sort out the normal and abnormal results so that I could focus on the abnormal results first and later in the day when I had more time I would look at the remainder.

Rank 5: C

It is important that I make referrals expediently. In this case, I saw the patient that morning and had assured myself it was safe for this patient to be seen routinely. Therefore it would not be harmful to the patient if I left this task to last. I would also ensure that the secretaries were aware that this referral did not need to be typed immediately and could wait until Monday morning if necessary.

Reflective question: What would you do differently next time?

I found task E the most difficult to rank. It is a personal issue and without further information, it was difficult to know how much it would affect me. I felt that I should call my brother quite promptly to find out what had happened as otherwise I would be worrying about her and this could affect my concentration and my ability to work effectively and this could compromise clinical care. It is very important that I recognize the impact of my personal life on my working day and that I do what I can to minimize the effect on my clinical work.

Practice example 1

You are a Foundation Year 2 doctor on-call for medicine

A. Mr Smith has been referred by A&E. He has been admitted with DKA (diabetic ketoacidosis), is on insulin and fluids and is stable.

B. You are bleeped by the ward to come and reinsert a cannula.

C. You are informed that Mr Reed, an inpatient with metastatic lung cancer, is in pain.

D. You need to complete your diary card and hand it in before the end of shift.

E. A local GP is trying to get hold of you to discuss Miss Gray, who was discharged by your team yesterday.

Rank:

Rank:

Rank:

Rank:

Rank:

Key points for practice example 1

- There are potentially two urgent clinical problems – the patient with DKA and the patient in pain. These should be your priority.
- Think about other help available to you – other members of your team might be free to assist you, if it is during the day there may be a palliative care team who could review Mr Reed urgently, someone from the diabetic team might be able to see Mr Smith. Is anyone else available who can do cannulae?
- Miss Gray's GP may simply require further information which the administration staff can provide or may wish to speak to you as she is unwell or there is a problem with her medication. Is anyone else available to ring him and maybe fax him a discharge summary.

Practice example 2

You are a Foundation Year 2 doctor doing an obstetrics and gynaecology post.

A. Your registrar would like to speak to you regarding the rota. One of your colleagues has phoned in sick for tomorrow.
B. You have a missed call from your sister on your mobile.
C. You have been referred a woman from A&E who is 6 weeks pregnant and has had vaginal bleeding for the last few hours. Her observations are stable.
D. A patient on the gynaecology ward needs fluids writing up.
E. A patient has been brought to labour ward. She is 33 weeks pregnant and has abdominal pain.

Rank:

Rank:

Rank:

Rank:

Rank:

Key points for practice example 2

- There are two potentially urgent clinical problems – the patient with PV bleeding may have an ectopic, the patient with abdominal pain may have an abruption. Think about what other help you have available to you in dealing with these two.
- Your sister may ring you every day and in this case a missed call would not bother you, but maybe she knows not to call you at work and would only do so if it is urgent. In this case, this is likely to affect your concentration and performance at work and it would be important to deal with this quickly. But not if patient safety is at risk.
- It is important that rotas are covered for good clinical care and if a locum is required, it is more likely one will be found if the staffing department is given adequate time.

Practice example 3

You are a hospital junior doctor on-call for paediatrics.

- A. There is a 3-month-old baby in A&E with a fever.
- B. Three medical students have arrived. You are due to teach them now.
- C. Your registrar needs your help to do a lumbar puncture on a 4-year-old girl.
- D. You are due to present your audit tomorrow and have not yet written the presentation.
- E. Your partner has left you a message. He has crashed his car, but says he is alright.

Rank:

Rank:

Rank:

Rank:

Rank:

Key points for practice example 3

- Show you recognize urgent clinical issues – baby with fever and deal with this promptly.
- Think of alternatives for the medical students rather than face–face teaching, maybe they could research a particular topic and present it to you later, they could help you manage the baby with a fever or help your registrar with the LP.
- Do not automatically put your partner to the bottom of the list. Although they have let you know they are fine, this is likely to be on your mind, until you have been reassured by speaking to them.

Practice example 4

You are a Foundation Year 2 doctor in general practice:

   A. You need to arrange some holiday insurance. You are due to fly out tomorrow.

   B. A pharmaceutical representative is waiting outside and would like to see you about a new inhaler.

   C. Your GP supervisor has left you a message – he would like to speak to you about a patient you saw this morning.

D. A receptionist rings you – Mr Taylor is on the phone requesting a home visit, but she is concerned as he seems to be having difficulty breathing.

E. The local pharmacy would like to speak to you. There is a problem with one of your prescriptions.

Rank:

Rank:

Rank:

Rank:

Rank:

Key points for practice example 4

- Deal with the urgent clinical issues first – Mr Taylor might have severe COPD and always have SOB (shortness of breath), but without further information this is potentially an urgent clinical problem and you may find after speaking to him that it is more appropriate that an ambulance is called rather than home wait for a home visit.

- Think about other help available to you. You are in a GP practice – there is usually a member of staff who deals with prescriptions and the local pharmacies. It may be that you can delegate this task to them or they could be obtaining more information before you are able to deal with it to make it easier for you.

SECTION G

Stage 4: Offer and allocation

Stage 4 is the final stage of the GP specialty training entry process and basically gives the overall outcome. You will receive this by email. This section addresses what happens next if you are successful or unsuccessful at achieving entry into GP specialty training.

13 Successful application to GP specialty training

Jasdeep Gill

Introduction

If successful, the deanery will email you an offer. Hooray! Give yourself a pat on the back! This offer will state allocation to a GP programme within the deanery and area based on your ranked preferences and performance, but will be subject to the usual pre-employment checks. If you are a Foundation Year 2 doctor, the offer will also be subject to you being awarded the FACD 5.2. You will need to forward this to the deanery once you get it. This is an essential document and you cannot progress from foundation training without it.

Remember you will have only 48 hours to accept the offer, excluding bank holidays and weekends. You should act on the email straightaway rather than wait. The deanery may set a date after which the offer will expire and be regarded as declined if you have not confirmed that you accept the offer. All your hard work will have gone to waste if you get this far and don't remember to accept the offer.

If you are waiting for the outcome of an application to Core Medical Training or Psychiatry (in England) and you wish to 'hold' the GP specialty training offer, then you should inform the deanery of this within the 48 hours. If you wish to decline the offer for whatever reason, it is considered good practice to reply with confirmation of this so that programmes can be allocated to another applicant if appropriate.

Your offer will expire and be deemed to have been declined if you do not confirm your acceptance.

Your employing hospital will then contact you with details of the rotations available which you need to rank in order of preference. These are then allocated based on your performance during the GP entry process. Sometimes, it can take quite some time for your hospital to contact you. Do not panic! They are likely to be very busy and inundated with work during this busy time. Do not harass your deanery because they will not be able to give you information, but if you need to contact someone then your hospital should be your first port of call.

You can then breathe a sigh of relief and look forward to the start of your GP speciality training!

Overview of what to expect once you start your GP training

Come August and the start of your GP training, you will meet plenty of friendly new faces. Hopefully, you will have received information about when your GP training days are and who your educational and clinical supervisors are. You will need to have at least two meetings per rotation with each of your supervisors and the onus is on you to organize these.

You will have a GP e-portfolio via the Royal College of General Practitioners (RCGP) website in which you must record all your meetings, learning log, professional development plan, reflection on experiences and DOPS, miniCEX and CBDs. The e-portfolio is a key tool during your GP specialty training. Log into this as soon as possible so you become familiar with it. You should aim to make an entry into your e-portfolio at least once a week, if not on a daily basis. It is vital that you work with the e-portfolio and keep it up to date, because it will be reviewed at the end of each year for your ARCP (Annual Review of Competence Progression).

Sometimes trainees can be unhappy with the rotation they are allocated. These may be fixed by the deanery and non-negotiable depending on local rules. It may be worth discussing with your local programme director if you have a particular problem. Irrespective of the components of your rotation, it is what you take from it that will round you as a better GP. The GP NPS for the entry process features the key themes, and these are what you should continue to focus on developing during your GP ST programme.

Above all, you should enjoy your GP specialty training! Aim to fulfil the requirements within the GP curriculum, but also aim to make the most of learning about areas that specifically interest you.

14 Unsuccessful application to GP specialty training

Jasdeep Gill

Introduction

Do not despair if you are unsuccessful at gaining entry into GP specialty training. Undoubtedly, you will have worked hard and will be upset. But do not despair as there are several options available to you.

You could try again. A process of local and national clearing will take place for applicants who were considered suitable for GP specialty training, but did not rank highly enough for the number of posts available within that deanery. These applicants will be considered on a ranked basis for any allocations that are declined locally within the deanery.

A 'round 2' process occurs for any unfilled posts, which are advertised nationally on the GP NRO website and applicants are invited to apply for any remaining vacancies. Bear in mind that not all deaneries have vacancies remaining, particularly the 'popular' deaneries such as London and Oxford. Both existing applicants and new applicants can apply to round 2. New applicants will need to ensure that they meet the entry criteria and have all the necessary documentation as outlined in Chapter 4 and submit an application. Existing applicants must not reapply, instead you have to ask for your application to be reinstated by contacting the GP NRO.

If you are an existing applicant who was unsuccessful because you did not provide the satisfactory evidence of foundation competency achievement, or because you failed at the stage 3 selection centre, then you will be considered in the round 2 process. You will be given the opportunity to attend a selection centre again, and provide the necessary evidence of competence. However, if you were unsuccessful because you failed the stage 2 situational judgement test then you cannot be considered in the round 2 process and will have to wait until the next cohort applies the following year.

Your primary concern is likely to be that you need to be employed come August. You should discuss your alternative options with your clinical and educational supervisors. These include an extension to your existing contract, locum shifts or research.

Re-evaluate your strategy

Think about why you may have been unsuccessful at gaining entry. Do not be negatively critical and think 'I'm useless and not good enough to be a GP' nor have the approach of 'it's the system, not me'. Start back at the beginning and reflect upon the entire entry process. You are likely to receive feedback if unsuccessful and you should take heed of this feedback, particularly if you reapply.

You should take a step back and reassess your choices. Perhaps general practice is not for you or indeed where your heart is? Reconsider where you see yourself in the future and which specialties appeal to you the most. If GP really is where you want to be, then chin up and try again. We wish you the best of luck!

SECTION H

Hot topics

15 Hot topics you should know about

Jasdeep Gill and Sukhjinder Nijjer

Introduction

This chapter focuses on key topics which are assessed during the GP entry process and will be relevant in your career. The following topics are likely to form questions or scenarios in several parts of the GP specialty training entry assessment. Therefore, a working knowledge of the following topics is required.

Clinical governance

Clinical governance is a framework through which organizations are accountable for continuously improving the quality of their services and safeguarding high standards of care by creating an environment in which excellence in clinical care will flourish.

Department of Health

Clinical governance is an integral part of the day to day responsibilities of a doctor. The key elements of clinical governance have traditionally been described using 'seven pillars' (see the box below). During your medical career so far you will have had direct experience of some of these pillars such as audit, training and research. If you think very carefully, it is possible to place all your daily activities within the seven pillars and you should do this in preparation for stages 2 and 3. For a GP, all seven pillars are vitally important both in their clinical work and for the smooth running of their practice.

Seven pillars of clinical governance

Audit

Risk management

Clinical effectiveness and research

Education and training

Patient and public involvement

IT and using information

Staffing and staff management

Audit

The process of clinical audit involves the review of current clinical practice against set standards of care to allow improvements in services and help maintain quality of care. If the set standard is not reached then the auditor needs to identify changes to be implemented. Once these changes have been implemented, the audit should be reconducted in order to complete the audit cycle, as illustrated in Figure 15.1. A common pitfall is that many applicants never complete an audit cycle because it is never reaudited. This could reflect negatively on an applicant if several audits have been started but none completed. You should aim to reaudit or have some follow-up knowledge of the audits which you have conducted so that you can state this in the stage 1 on-line application.

An audit-related question could easily appear within the simulation exercise or the SJT assessment. Refer back to scenarios from your experience and to the worked examples in this book and think about how you would deal with such a question.

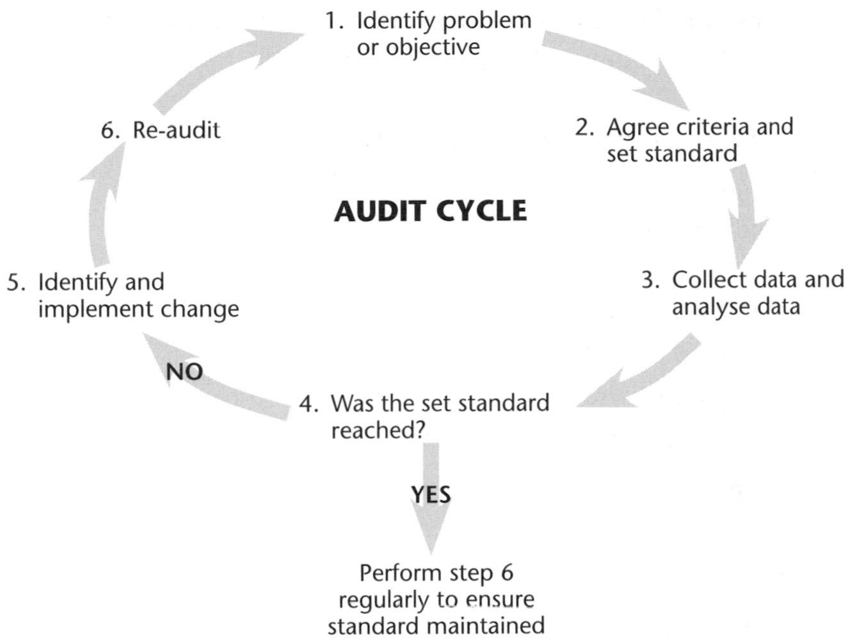

1. Identify problem
   or objective

6. Re-audit

2. Agree criteria and
   set standard

AUDIT CYCLE

5. Identify and
   implement change

3. Collect data and
   analyse data

NO

4. Was the set standard
   reached?

YES

Perform step 6
regularly to ensure
standard maintained

Figure 15.1 Audit cycle

Risk management

Inevitably, things can and do go wrong! This pillar of clinical governance focuses on having robust systems to understand, reflect upon and minimize the risks. It incorporates important issues such as reporting significant adverse events to allow a stepwise analysis to be conducted, complying with protocols such as discarding sharps, handling and learning from complaints. Regular practice meetings often assist with such matters, but it is necessary to promote a blame-free culture and encourage input from the multidisciplinary team.

As a GP, you will need to reflect upon and learn from adverse events to help improve your work and reduce future risks. Unlike hospital-based doctors, GPs can feel isolated during adverse events and therefore need a good structure of review and support. This means risk management issues are frequently tested during the entry process.

The simulation exercise could incorporate issues surrounding risk management. For example, you could be asked to discuss a recent significant event analysis with the practice manager and fellow partner in the simulation exercise. Knowing how to interact with your colleagues to achieve the best outcome is essential. Identifying all the factors that lead to the error or risk and discussing them in turn, while being open to your colleagues' ideas is essential. Refer back to scenarios from your experience and to the worked examples in this book and think about how you would deal with such a question.

Clinical effectiveness and research

This involves practising evidence-based medicine, conducting research to enhance the evidence base, and implementing national guidelines such as NICE and National Service Frameworks. The aim is to provide optimal clinical care for patients. You may have conducted research at medical school and you may have helped write clinical guidelines at work. Many doctors say they are following 'evidence-based medicine' without truly understanding the complexity of applying research performed in highly selected populations, to the patient in hand.

Questions relating to clinical effectiveness and research are likely to form part of the stage 2 assessment. For example, MCQ questions relating to the management of patients based on national guidelines are often asked. Commonly tested areas are asthma and hypertension management.

Education and training

This relates to continuous professional development (CPD) and highlights the importance of lifelong learning for a doctor. It has gained increased attention over recent years with the introduction of appraisals and revalidation. The ever-changing nature of medicine and the generalist approach of a GP mean that on-going education and lifelong learning is mandatory. This should be targeted or focused learning which is informed by performance feedback and reflection to identify the doctor's learning needs. A

GP must identify their own learning needs and must maintain a portfolio of learning activities and their application.

All relevant courses and exams will need to be entered on the application form in stage 1. The types of courses and exams undertaken by a candidate can help demonstrate commitment to the GP specialty. Think carefully which courses to undertake to support your application.

Patient and public involvement

This involves obtaining regular feedback from patients and public to help improve the quality of care and tailor services to meet their needs. Feedback can be obtained via patient forums as local involvement networks (LINks) and feedback questionnaires on a local or national scale.

Your knowledge of such areas could be tested in a simulation exercise. For example, a scenario may involve discussion with a colleague about a recent patient satisfaction questionnaire in which the patients rated accessibility to the practice as 'poor'. You could discuss the financial implications of this, the need to organise a patient forum to obtain more information about this and ideas on how to improve the service. Refer to scenarios from your experience and to the worked examples in this book and consider how you would deal with such a question.

IT and using information

The computerization of UK general practice is almost universal and in fact, predates hospital computer systems. General practice has gradually adopted computerization due to a variety of government incentives and reforms, social expectations and administrative benefits. There are various software systems in use and they cover various aspects of practice from booking appointments to audit. All systems must be approved by the Department of Health.

This pillar of clinical governance addresses the need to ensure patient data are up to date and that appropriate data protection measures are in place. It also highlights the use of IT in aiding service development, by measuring quality of outcomes and conducting audits, for example. Furthermore, it incorporates the use of Choose and Book services and electronic prescribing. Your awareness of this could be tested in the simulation exercise.

Staffing and staff management

It is useful for GPs to have a working knowledge of staffing issues, such as recruitment and staff management, because practices do not have a large human resources department like hospitals to deal with such matters.

It is very difficult to keep on top of the frequent changes in employment law and this is a particularly complex area. It covers areas such as employment contracts, pay, pensions, notice periods, working hours, annual leave, maternity/paternity leave, discrimination, unfair dismissal and so on. If in any doubt, you should contact your defence union for advice. Often the practice manager and a nominated GP within a practice take the lead on staffing issues. However, all GPs need an awareness of areas such as maintaining good working conditions, addressing underperformance and organizing adequate cover in the event of staff absences.

This could be tested in the simulation exercise. For example, if you are given a scenario which requires discussion of an underperforming colleague. Refer back to the worked examples in this book and think about how you would deal with such a question.

Fitness to drive

Patients with certain medical conditions may not satisfy the medical standards required for safe driving. Patients with a driving licence who do not meet driving standards have a legal duty to inform the DVLA (Driver and Vehicle Licensing Agency). When considering a patient's fitness to drive, it needs to be done in the context of their type of driving licence.

There are two types of driving licence: group 1 and group 2. Group 1 is the 'ordinary' licence for driving a private car or motorcycle. Group 2 licences are for driving heavy goods vehicles (HGV) or passenger carrying vehicles (PCV), such as buses and taxis. There is an extensive document produced by the DVLA on current medical standards of fitness to drive and you should familiarize yourself with this via their website. It includes information about both group 1 and 2 licence holders and it changes regularly. For your day-to-day practice, you should remember to check it regularly. For the GP entry process, you should be familiar with its rules for common conditions.

When handling fitness to drive scenarios, you should first ensure that the patient understands that they cannot drive because their condition can impair their ability to drive and cause danger to themselves and the public. You must inform the patient of their legal duty to inform the DVLA. If the patient continues to drive, you must make a reasonable effort to persuade the patient to stop driving and remind them to notify the DVLA. Unfortunately, if the patient still continues to drive or cannot be persuaded to stop driving, then it is up to you to disclose this to the medical adviser at the DVLA. This disclosure is made in the interests of public safety and is a recognized exemption to your duty to patient confidentiality. Prior to informing the DVLA, you must inform the patient and subsequently write to the patient confirming that disclosure to the DVLA has been made.

If the situation involves an incompetent patient, with dementia for example, then you should inform the DVLA immediately on their behalf. You also need to ensure that your consultations and advice are fully documented in the notes. If you are in any doubt, you should seek advice from your defence union.

The DVLA will then send the patient a medical questionnaire and obtain their consent to request more information from their doctor. Once the DVLA has reviewed the patient's case against the medical standards of fitness to drive, they will make the decision of whether to issue, revoke or refuse a licence. If a patient's licence is revoked or refused, they will be given an explanation of why this decision was made and circumstances in which they could reapply. They will also receive information about their right to appeal, which will be handled by the courts.

Patients with any condition or disability that may cause danger to the public if they were to drive, must be advised not to drive and that they have a legal duty to inform the DVLA.

This is a very common theme for the GP entry process. The SJT in stage 2 commonly tests the theoretical knowledge of the DVLA guidelines in the clinical problem-solving paper and also tests your application of theory alongside legal and ethical issues in the professional dilemmas. The commonly encountered questions in stage 2 relate to neurological, cardiovascular, diabetic and sleep disorders – although it is not unheard of for questions to crop up relating to other disorders. So be prepared! You should refer to the up-to-date medical standards of fitness to drive guidelines or summary from the DVLA website.

It could also be tested in stage 3 within the simulation exercise. For example, a patient could be making a complaint because disclosure to the DVLA was made against their wishes and supposedly not handled correctly by one of the salaried GPs. Another example may be that an incident occurred where a patient continued to drive despite warnings not to. In this scenario, the patient drove into a tree causing a fractured femur but without harming anybody else. Your task may involve deciding to have a significant event analysis meeting.

Alternatively, in a patient simulation exercise, you may encounter a taxi driver who is consulting following a STEMI (ST segment elevation myocardial infarction). This could be a complex scenario and require the doctor to deal with issues around discussing a new diagnosis, as well as informing the patient of his legal duty as a taxi driver to inform the DVLA and to stop driving for at least 6 months. The consultation would require knowledge of clinical guidelines, secondary prevention and information about support groups to ensure that the patient is treated holistically.

Gifts

GPs are often given gifts from their patients as a way of saying thank you for treating them or a family member. These often come in the form of a tasty box of chocolates or a small food hamper, for example at Christmas. However, sometimes the gift can be more substantial. The GMC is clear in their guidance that doctors must not encourage gifts or money from patients.

You must not encourage patients to give, lend or bequeath money or gifts that will directly or indirectly benefit you.

General Medical Council (GMC)

This could be assessed in stage 2 or 3 or the GP entry process. Each scenario will require your personal judgement as to whether or not the gift is appropriate and acceptable. This can be difficult to do. First, you should consider why the patient is giving the gift. If the doctor has asked for the gift, then it is most certainly incorrect. If the patient seems to have an ulterior motive, such as trying to bribe the doctor for 'better' care or seduce the doctor, then again it is incorrect. Then, you should consider the gift itself. If the value of the gift is too high or disproportionate, then you should question accepting it. Finally, you should consider the implications of accepting or refusing the gift. For example, refusing a box of chocolates from a well-known patient is likely to cause them offence and may even upset the doctor–patient relationship. Whether or not you accept the gift, you should explain your reasoning clearly to avoid any misunderstandings.

Consent

All procedures, examination and treatment require valid consent. This may be implied, verbal or written. For consent to be legally valid, the following must occur:

- The patient must have capacity to give consent.
- It must be an informed decision.
- Consent must be given voluntarily.

Here, we will look at these components of consent. The terms 'capacity' and 'competence' are often used interchangeably. It is judged clinically and a patient may have capacity for one decision, but not for another.

For a patient to have capacity and be deemed competent, they must understand and believe what is being proposed; understand its benefits, risks and alternatives; understand the consequences of not having the intervention; retain the information for sufficient time to use it and weigh it in balance to arrive at a decision. Capacity is decision- and time-specific, so it should be assessed every time consent is sought.

For patients who lack capacity, no person can consent to medical treatment on behalf of another adult. Doctors may treat a patient lacking capacity, without consent, under common law providing the treatment/procedure is necessary and in the patient's best interests. Relatives should be involved in discussions, but cannot make the final decision.

All adults (over 16 years of age) are assumed to have capacity to give consent unless proven otherwise. The situation is more complex in children. A competent child must demonstrate understanding of what is proposed, its possible complications and consequences of not having the proposed treatment. This is referred to as 'Gillick' competence. If Gillick competent, the child can consent without the need for parental permission or knowledge. However, if the child were to refuse, then a parent or court can authorise the proposed care in the child's best interests. In a non-competent child, only a parent or person with parental responsibility can agree to or refuse the proposed care.

A special set of guidelines apply when considering the use of contraception in those under 16 years of age. These are referred to as the Fraser guidelines or criteria. If a patient meets the Fraser criteria, a doctor can provide contraceptive advice and treatment without needing parental consent. The Fraser criteria are as follows: that the young person understands the doctor's advice, cannot be persuaded to inform their parents, is likely to have sexual intercourse irrespective of contraception, that their physical or mental health may suffer without the contraception and that the doctor is acting in their best interests.

In emergencies, if the patient is competent, consent should be gained. If the patient cannot give consent, for example if unconscious, then emergency treatment and procedures should be performed in their best interests.

Remember, consent is a dynamic situation and the patient can withdraw consent at any time. Consent is not purely a signature on paper – an ill-informed patient or one who is coerced has not given legally valid consent. Furthermore, a competent patient can refuse any procedure or treatment for any reason, rational or otherwise, even if such a choice is fatal for the patient. To proceed against a patient's wishes constitutes battery. Withdrawal of consent should not prejudice the patient's care: just because the patient has declined one treatment option, does not mean they cannot have any treatment.

Consent issues may be tested in stage 3 during the simulation exercise. Avoid jargon during your discussion and do not make assumptions. A patient's true understanding can differ wildly from superficial smiles and nods. Give information in small chunks and repeatedly check their understanding. Remind them that they can refuse the procedure and never coerce the patient to have it. If they do refuse, offer them the next best alternative. You should offer a patient information leaflet at the end of your simulation exercise to help reinforce the points you have discussed and you could invite the patient to return if they have any further questions having read the leaflet.

Always seek the latest guidance on consent, capacity and controversial areas, such as treating minors or those without capacity. Your defence union may provide you with helpful advice and information.

Issues surrounding consent could be assessed in stage 2 within the professional dilemma paper. For example, you could be asked to rank the responses given for a 58-year-old patient who is refusing treatment for breast cancer.

Confidentiality

Maintaining confidentiality is an essential element of the doctor–patient relationship. There are several legal viewpoints which safeguard this right to confidentiality, such as the Common Law of Confidentiality and the Data Protection Act.

However, there are exceptional circumstances in which confidentiality may be breeched:

- **Public interest:** the benefit of disclosure must outweigh the patient's personal interest of maintaining confidentiality, for example to the DVLA.
- **Danger or emergencies:** where disclosure may be necessary to prevent or reduce a serious/imminent threat to life or health of the individual or another person, for example in child protection issues.
- **Statutory requirement:** legal requirement for disclosure, for example notifiable disease reporting is statutory.
- **Adverse drug reactions:** requires reporting to the Medicines and Healthcare Products Regulatory Agency.
- **Court or tribunal request:** if you are ordered by a court judge to disclose information. However, remember that you must not breach confidentiality when discussing with solicitors, police officers or others.

In the exceptional circumstance when you may need to breach confidentiality, you must have appropriate justification and have at least informed the patient of the disclosure. All other circumstances require the patient's explicit consent.

Child protection

As a GP, you will be in daily contact with children and in many cases directly responsible for their care. Child protection and safeguarding children has become an increasingly important part of doctors' training and roles. If you are concerned about a child's well-being or suspect they may be at risk of abuse or neglect, then you must act upon these concerns in accordance with local and national protocols.

A child can suffer abuse or neglect either from direct harm or from a failure to prevent harm occurring. Child abuse and neglect can have significant detrimental effects on a child's health, development or life.

Key types of child abuse

Physical abuse

Emotional abuse

Sexual abuse

Neglect

You are likely to encounter questions relating to child protection in the stage 2 assessment. For example, you may be asked to rank certain options relating to a question about a 15-year-old girl who has been found to have an ectopic pregnancy. This type of scenario would require you to consider if the patient is Gillick competent or not, was it consensual intercourse, who was the partner and what age. If the patient was under the age of 13 years, then your considerations would be different because the law clearly states that anyone under the age of 13 years is not competent to consent to sexual activity. Therefore, it would constitute rape so the police and social services would have to be involved. If the partner was 23 years old, then you would have to consider child protection and safety issues for the pregnant girl.

All doctors working with children and adults who are in contact with children, must be able to recognize signs that a child could be at risk of abuse or neglect and must be familiar with local child protection procedures.

It is also important for you to remember the impact of illness in the parent or guardian looking after a child and how this may impact on the child safety and well-being. For example, this may be relevant for an alcoholic patient who is drinking a bottle of vodka a day and living with her 2-year-old daughter. Refer back to the worked examples in the book and consider how you would handle such a scenario.

Complaints

Complaints in the NHS are common and general practice is no exception. Despite knowing this fact, it does not make dealing with a complaint against you easier. It can be stressful and it is tempting to put your head in the sand and avoid managing it. A constructive way of dealing with a complaint is to view it as a learning experience. By doing so, you are not belittling the complaint in any way, but instead your approach to it will be more open and constructive. It is also worthwhile talking to senior colleagues about the situation who may be able to help or offer advice.

Since April 2009, there has been a change to the NHS complaints process. The new complaints procedure consists of a two-tier framework, as opposed to three in the previous system. The changes were introduced to make the process more straightforward and streamlined with less time delay through adherence to bureaucratic processes.

The two-tier framework consists of 'local resolution' in the first instance. This allows patients to complain to the practice or *Patient Advice and Liaison Services (PALS)*, or to the PCT directly if they do not wish to complain to the organization against which they have a complaint. The majority of complaints should be managed effectively at this stage and reach resolution. However, if the patient is unsatisfied with the outcome, they can proceed to the next step and request a review by the ombudsman which represents the second tier of the framework.

There are several ways of dealing with a complaint. We have devised a helpful mnemonic to help you remember the fundamental points: 'COMPLAINTS'.

The 'COMPLAINTS' technique to handling local complaints

C	Clarify the complaint
O	Offer apology and objective investigation
M	Meeting
P	People and practice
L	Learn from it
A	Accurate record keeping
I	Inform and update the patient at all times
N	Next steps if no resolution – ombudsman
T	Take a step back
S	Stress – don't!

Clarify the complaint

Aim to establish the patient's exact concern and complaint. Sometimes this can be difficult because complaints are often multifactorial and the patient may have sent a lengthy letter listing many issues which are not always directly related to you. It is also helpful to establish the patient's expectations early on to help guide resolution.

Offer apology and objective investigation

Always apologise at the earliest opportunity. An apology is not an admission of guilt; instead it can help diffuse the situation. You should offer an objective investigation into all complaints. This can be difficult, particularly if the complaint contains personal or direct comments against you. Try not to take the criticism or complaint personally as this can lead to an unsympathetic approach, which would only worsen matters. Sometimes it is worthwhile if another person, often practice manager or a colleague, deals with the formalities of the complaint.

Meetings

Arrange meetings to discuss the complaint with those involved and colleagues. A meeting with the patient will also need to be arranged. All meetings should be conducted in a professional manner with a 'no blame' culture adopted. Consider the use of conciliation early, involving an independent mediator. Either party can ask for conciliation, but both parties have to agree to it. The two parties are brought together and discuss matters with a conciliator present. It is a non-threatening and helpful way to explain matters and ensure the parties are listening to each other.

People and practice

Deciding which people to involve is an important step because some complaints may be of a sensitive nature or may cause a lot of disruption in small practices. If the complaint is of a serious nature involving a clinician, it is also important to decide if they should continue practising while the complaint is under investigation and unresolved.

Learn from it

Complaints should be viewed in a constructive light and used as a learning experience. You should personally reflect upon what you have learnt from the situation and what you will do differently in future. If the complaint relates to a systems error, then lessons should be learnt about how this can be avoided and what should be changed in order to help.

Accurate record keeping

This is important in all aspects of medicine, more so with the increasing medicolegal culture in society. The complaint, acknowledgement and response must be in writing. Documentation or minutes should be made for all conversations or meetings conducted and of any actions or agreement reached. The last thing you would want is another complaint about how the complaint was handled and then no supporting evidence for your case.

Inform and update the patient at all times

Poor communication and misunderstandings are a common reason for complaints in the first place. Therefore, you should do your utmost to ensure these mistakes are not repeated. Sometimes, an unavoidable delay can occur while dealing with a complaint, such as unexpected sickness or absence of a key individual. The patient should be informed of this and how it may impact the time-frame or resolution of their complaint.

Next steps if no resolution

The new two-tier complaints procedure means that the next step is the ombudsman.

Take a step back

Think about and analyse why local resolution did not occur. The majority of complaints result in local resolution, so it is worthwhile considering what was different in this case. Consider factors relating to the complaint itself, the practice complaint policy, attitudes towards complaints and how they are managed.

Stress – Don't!

That is easier said than done, but it is important that you do not allow it to effect your own well-being or that of your other patients. Any complaint, at any stage in your career, is stressful. You should seek support from family, colleagues or external agencies early on to help.

You are likely to encounter handling complaints in the professional dilemma paper of stage 2 and in the stage 3, during the simulation exercise. For example, an angry patient comes to see you to complain because her 15-year-old daughter was prescribed the oral contraceptive pill the previous week. This would assess your communication, coping under pressure, empathy and sensitivity skills. It would also assess your knowledge of professional integrity and awareness of issues such as consent and confidentiality. As another example, you may be asked to discuss a recent complaint against a nurse in the practice who administered the MMR vaccine to a baby, whose mother subsequently denies giving consent. Refer back to the worked examples in this book and consider how you would deal with such a scenario. Also consider which of the NPS items are being assessed and how best you can demonstrate them within the scenario.

Index

Note: page numbers in **bold** refer to diagrams.